Advance Praise for *Autism Adulthood*

"There is a huge need for books to help individuals with autism make the transition to adulthood. . . . I highly recommend *Autism Adulthood* for parents and teachers who are guiding individuals in the middle range within the broad autism spectrum." —Temple Grandin, author of *The Autistic Brain* and *Thinking in Pictures*

"In this book, like her others, the wonderful Susan Senator gives voice to those who are too often voiceless—folks with ASD who seek what they deserve—lives of purpose and possibilities." —Ron Suskind, Pulitzer Prize–winning journalist and bestselling author of *Life Animated: A Story of Sidekicks, Heroes, and Autism*

"In her frank and deeply touching new book, *Autism Adulthood*, Susan Senator shares the intimate details of her journey with her son, Nat, as he takes his first steps toward maturity in a society that offers few resources for people on the spectrum after they 'age out' of the meager level of services provided to school-age children. She faces the big issues—housing, employment, relationships with siblings, finding trustworthy caregivers—head-on, and offers practical strategies for giving young autistic people the best chance to lead happy, safe, and secure lives, mapping a pathway to the future that offers autistic people and their families real hope, rather than false hopes built on misguided promises of a cure. By doing so she offers a blueprint for a world in which people at every point on the spectrum are treated as fellow citizens who deserve respect and the ability to make choices, rather than as puzzles to be solved by the next medical breakthrough." —Steve Silberman, author of *NeuroTribes: The Legacy of Autism and the Future of Neurodiversity*

"From the introduction, *Autism Adulthood: Strategies and Insights for a Fulfilling Life* will bring you to that dark place parents of young adults with autism fear. But just as quickly, Susan offers practical advice through storytelling and concise, how-to strategies that will leave you feeling optimistic, hopeful, and back in control—all any of us can ask for. A thoroughly readable and important book."
—Arthur Fleischmann, author of *Carly's Voice: Breaking Through Autism*

"*Autism Adulthood* is a book I will be recommending to every autism parent I know. Senator is as warm as she is wise, as thoughtful as she is knowledgeable, as compassionate as she is informative. Her rallying cry of, "All we can do is love each other," will resound in any parent's heart. Senator loves fiercely—which means she does everything she can to ensure the best life and future for her adult child with autism. This book will inspire the rest of us to do the same for ours." —Claire LaZebnik, coauthor of *Overcoming Autism*, with Dr. Lynn Kern Koegel

"Susan's book is a must-read not only autism parents but for disability parents in general." —Laura Shumaker, author of *A Regular Guy: Growing Up with Autism* and writer for the *San Francisco Chronicle*

AUTISM
ADULTHOOD

Also by Susan Senator
Making Peace with Autism
An Autism Mom's Survival Guide

AUTISM ADULTHOOD

STRATEGIES

AND

INSIGHTS

FOR A

FULFILLING

LIFE

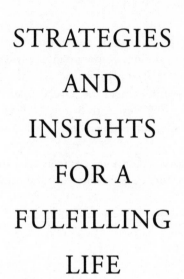

SUSAN SENATOR

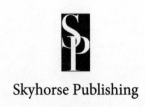

Skyhorse Publishing

Skyhorse Publishing books may be purchased in bulk at special discounts for sales promotion, corporate gifts, fund-raising, or educational purposes. Special editions can also be created to specifications. For details, contact the Special Sales Department, Skyhorse Publishing, 307 West 36th Street, 11th Floor, New York, NY 10018 or info@skyhorsepublishing.com.

Skyhorse® and Skyhorse Publishing® are registered trademarks of Skyhorse Publishing, Inc.®, a Delaware corporation.

Visit our website at www.skyhorsepublishing.com.

10 9 8 7 6 5 4 3 2 1

Library of Congress Cataloging-in-Publication Data is available on file.

Print ISBN: 978-151070-423-7
Ebook ISBN: 978-151070-424-4

Printed in the United States of America

Dedicated to
Ned, Nat, Max, and Ben

ACKNOWLEDGMENTS

ALL OF US NEED others to show us the way. And so I need to acknowledge my "others," those autistic adults who helped me understand to the degree that I could, what their lives are like. First of all, Nat. I hope he knows how much he has taught me about life, love, and autism. I have told him again and again that I write about him and that he helps others by letting me use his story. I tell him: "I write about you because you have autism, and people want to know about that. And because you do such a good job at home, and at work, helping out." He's on the forefront of developmentally delayed autistics who are making their way in the world.

I also want to thank the autistic activists and bloggers, some of whom I connected with online: Camille, who runs the *Autism Diva*; Prometheus, who runs *A Photon in the Darkness*; and Landon, creator of the blogazine thAutcast.com. There are also the autistic self-advocates I've met at Autistic Self-Advocacy Network meetings and parties: Ivan, Ari, Lydia, Kate, and Michael, all of whom taught me that there is no such thing as high-functioning autism, in that verbal or nonverbal speech are never an indicator of the intensity of one's challenges.

Also thank you to the community of autism writers, bloggers, and thinkers who have inspired me: Jess Wilson, Steve Silberman, Temple Grandin, Sean and Judy Barron, and to the families who gave me insight and told me their stories.

I have to honor my four gurus in autism adulthood services: Jeff Keilson, Mike Weiner, Elizabeth Sternberg, and Cathy Boyle. I know what I know because of you guys.

A shout-out to my community at Peet's Coffee Shop, who kept me company and full of coffee: Dave, Paul, Tim, and Marty. Deep appreciation to Emily Miles Terry, my writing buddy and longtime friend. So much gratitude to my publisher, Tony Lyons at Skyhorse; my editor, Lilly Golden; and my tough and dedicated agent, Diane Gedymin, who is like family to me. And finally, thank you to my family: Mom, Dad, Laura, and especially Nat, Max, and Ben, and to Ned, who is my soul mate, great love, and husband. I couldn't do it without all of you.

CONTENTS

Chapter Ten: I Can Never Die, and Other Myths

FOREWORD

by John Elder Robison, author of *Look Me in the Eye*

❧

Every autism parent I know has fantasized about the day their child grows up to be a software designer, or some other quirky independent professional. As parents and children grow older, the dream often changes to hoping the child can be independent. Finally, there is acceptance and the desire mainly for the child to be happy. We all want to be independent and do things for ourselves. But it does not always work out that way, particularly in our high-tech society. It's very hard for people with limited verbal skills to achieve independence in modern America. In years past, a non-speaking person could work with plants or animals, and be a contributing member of society without much language. Few such opportunities remain today. The job prospects for non-speaking adults are very limited, but they are improving.

And what if your child still needs care when he's an adult? We always hope that won't happen, but sometimes it does. For most families, the fact that both parents work outside the house complicates the situation. If the child needs help during the day, and mom and dad are gone, there is potential for crisis. That's a huge stressor for parents.

Susan Senator has written a touching and wise account of her son Nat's transition from the family home to supported living within the community. The book is accessible in that it reads like a memoir, yet it's practical too—filled with tips from other families who live with autism, and from professionals who work with our population. There have been quite a few memoirs from autism parents with small children. Many of those children were diagnosed within the past twenty years, and they are becoming adults today. A few will make a smooth transition to independent adulthood, but many won't. Susan's book speaks powerfully to the parents of those kids with more significant challenges.

We hope that our autistic children will be able to advocate for themselves. Many speaking autistic people can do this. Some autistic people who do not speak can still communicate their wants and needs through devices like the iPad. But there remain a number of autistic people whose cognitive and verbal challenges prevent them from communicating effectively or advocating, particularly in public. That portion of our population—partly because of their communication difficulty—is seldom seen or heard, and is often neglected. It's hard to know if we are meeting their needs, and what more we might do. Parents need help reading the cues, and knowing where to look for help. If you are an autism parent, and your child needs or may need extensive adult support, I highly recommend this book. I also recommend this book for clinicians and educators for its valuable insight into an oft-overlooked part of our community.

One day, we may learn how to help people like Nat communicate more effectively and even become more verbal. We may even figure out how to relieve cognitive impairments. But that day is not now, and waiting before we act helps no one. For now, we must do what Susan has done with such dedication for her son

Nat—work to give our children the best quality of life and the greatest degree of independence.

John Elder Robison is an autistic adult and advocate for people with neurological differences. He's the author of the international bestseller Look Me in the Eye, Be Different, Raising Cubby, *and* Switched On. *He's served on the Interagency Autism Coordinating Committee of the US Dept of Health and Human Services, committees for the National Institutes of Health (NIH) and the Centers for Disease Control and Prevention (CDC), and many other autism-related boards. He's co-founder of the TCS Auto Program (a school for teens with developmental challenges) and is the Neurodiversity Scholar in Residence at the College of William and Mary in Williamsburg, Virginia.*

PART I

CONSTRUCTING AUTISM ADULTHOOD

INTRODUCTION

Beginning at the End

THE OTHER DAY I had a vulnerable moment where I let myself imagine The End. If you're reading this, you know what I am referring to: the moment when I would no longer be here for my autistic son, Nat.

I don't like to talk about it. No one does. But we parents will only learn from each other if we talk about autism adulthood and what to do for our children in the long run.

So, there I am, lying down in a bed with old, thinning white hair and bony hands. Underweight for the first time in my life.

I'm falling into my last sleep. And there is Nat hovering nearby, glancing at me with overly bright eyes while moving around the room. Each time he looks over at me, he says, "Mommy will wake up." But of course, I can't. "Mommy will get up," he says again, his voice louder. Again and again, his tone sharpens and slices, but he cannot get through to me. He has never liked it when I nap. Sleep is for nighttime. And I have always been there for him, hovering in the background and, let's face it, in the foreground. I have had to be awake even while I sleep.

I have tried to cede him his independence. I divided myself, always keeping his sweet face—eyes still innocent despite his years—constantly at the forefront of my mind. Even though my husband, Ned, did a fine job with the scissors that evening so long ago in the maternity ward at Beth Israel Hospital in Boston, I have never thoroughly cut our cord.

(By the way, you may wonder, as I have, where the rest of my family is in this image of my deathbed—Ned and my other two sons, Max and Ben. My family is much bigger than Nat and me. Presumably they are nearby. But this picture in my head is just of Nat.)

I may hear his distress, faintly, but I can't do anything because I'm going wherever it is we go when we die. I can't help him. This is it, the moment I've dreaded for all of Nat's life. I have to leave him now. Someone else has to take care of him. Help him. Love him . . . He doesn't understand why Mommy won't get up.

I know, I know, this is so sad, and maybe even maudlin. Unrealistic. Besides, how many of us really get to be on a deathbed, saying our goodbyes when we are just so old and tired?

Still, it's what comes into my head sometimes—especially when I'm tired. I can't help it. Can you? Don't we all worry about our last moments and how to leave our children behind, so that they'll be okay?

That's why I'm writing this book. I need to help others who love someone with autism figure this out. Even if there are no definitive answers—and to tell you the truth, I'm not a big believer in definitive answers—I still want to find out everything I can for all those like me.

I wrote about my quest for a path to a fulfilling autism adulthood in the *Washington Post* in 2011:

Ever since Nat's birth back in the Autism Stone Age of 1989, I have had to be a Saber-Toothed Tiger Mother—or at least pretend to be one. From finding the right doctors to getting my town to do right by him, to also doing right by my other two sons, I have always had to be strong—or feign it. What to expect when you're not expecting autism? No one really had any answers—not then, not now. So it has always been up to my husband, Ned, and me.

I am told that I am special because I am Nat's mom. A saint. Chosen. But I'm not. I'm just a mother trying to raise my son to be the best he can be. The other thing I hear a lot is that Nat is an angel, closer to God than others, chosen to be here to teach me something. No, he's not. He is just a complex young man. He's neither a spiritual messenger nor a puzzle.

What happens in autism adulthood is the real puzzle. We're all tired of not knowing what to do—first, next, and last.

Helping Nat have a decent adult life is my family's greatest challenge with Nat—not Nat himself. We want him to have a life with something to do: a job, volunteer work. A place to live safely and cared for. Days with a rewarding rhythm. And so this is something I've been working on since he turned eighteen. Maybe earlier. Nat was working at Meals on Wheels by fourteen and at a fast food pizza chain by nineteen.

It has recently dawned on me that I am going to have to do more than act tough and tireless: I have to become what they say I am. Because I have to face the fact that no matter how hard I push, we still may not end up with all the pieces that compose what Nat or we, his parents, would deem a fulfilling life for him. If only there was a waiting list for adult life tasks like there are at the good autism schools. I know how to be on those. Still, I've tried for years to put together my vision for Nat: a home in the city, near mine; a great caregiver who would enrich his life. And every time I get close to succeeding, some piece or another does not fall into place. You can't get the funding for housing until you have a group. You can't get the group together until you have a house.

And so, on top of all the emotional upheaval, Nat's turning twenty-two is a catch-22. The funding is scarce, and the programs can be iffy because of it. And, as always, there's no one to ask for answers; every expert and professional has a different story. In the end, I'm figuring it out as I go; only now, I am no longer a young mother.

However, I am still Nat's mother; not really the tiger I'm supposed to be, but, uh, well, here it goes anyway: uh, roar.

Like most parents, I did not know how to deal with my autistic child's transition to adulthood. A disabled child's adulthood carries within it the ultimate fears about finding others to support his life: What will that life look like? Where will he live? And, of course, the one that haunts us the most—what will happen when I die?

Aside from the overwhelming specter of one's own death, there is a different sort of earthly fear in autism parenting. I think of it as the day-by-day anxiety about how your autistic loved one is living, in the form of Am I Doing This Right/Is He Happy? This worry is mixed in with certain worrisome practical considerations—the day-to-day life of your child and the long-term planning, e.g., the financing of adulthood, arranging trusts, finding staff and housing, daytime occupation, social life, healthcare.

This book is not going to cover the technical fiduciary matters like trusts, wills, or guardianships. Nor will you find information on what your particular state's laws and guidelines are for adult services. I will, however, refer you to lots of good places for that.

My book is more personal, more illustrative of what goes on when our adult children transition to their lives beyond school—what it looks like, feels like, and what we can do about it. Think of me as your autism pal who is experienced, immersed in the autism community for decades, and who would sit down with you over a coffee and help.

I am going to lay out a way for you to look at adulthood, through my own experience as a mom who is there right now, and from my years of being an author, researcher, speaker, and advocate in the field of autism. I will tell you my family's autism adulthood story theme by theme and in narrated snippets, and then provide you stories from others who are also there right now. Although I have changed some of the names and states of certain interviewees, the words and stories are true. Thus, I will give you a picture of what others' autism adult lives look like—from creating living situations to vocational fulfillment, to what it feels like to be on the autism spectrum. With real stories to go by, you will be able to project your loved one's own journey.

"People First" or "Autism Pride"?

You will find in reading this book that I interchange the terms "people with autism" with "autistic people." I am well aware of and respect the People First movement—the widespread effort to avoid defining someone by their disability (as in the latter example). A few of the people I interviewed specified that they preferred People First language, and I made sure I wrote their sections with that in mind. However, I also know of many people on the autism spectrum who *prefer* being referred to as "autistic." This group feels that they are indeed defined by their autism, that their personality is wrapped inextricably in autism, and, furthermore, that this is a point of pride. Hence, my solution is to use both terms interchangeably, because I see the value in both philosophies.

No doubt people will also note that I do not use the term "autism spectrum" too often, nor do I specifically distinguish between descriptions like high functioning, low functioning, Aspie, Aspergian, Aspergerian, pervasive developmental disordered, ASD (autism spectrum disorder), and just plain old autism. This is because the current DSM-V (Diagnostic and Statistical Manual of Mental Disorders, Fifth Edition) has eliminated many such divisions on the autism spectrum, focusing instead on descriptive designations and on determining possible *features* of autism (e.g. social, communicative, behavioral, sensory, or intellectual deficits) rather than labeling kinds of autism. Though there has been much discord among the medical, psychological, and autism communities about these changes in the DSM; many agree that terms such "high-functioning" or "low-functioning" autism are definitely outmoded, as they sprung from verbal competence or lack thereof. We now know that a person can be without verbal speech and still have the ability to express himself successfully. Likewise, someone with verbal speech and a very high IQ might be completely debilitated by depression or social, sensory, or behavioral challenges. So I, too, will stick to descriptions of skills and challenges to give you the full *human* picture of my subjects.

Speaking of the full human picture . . .

In my narrative, I try to avoid describing an autistic person's unusual actions as "behaviors," "stims," or "stereotypes." To me, these terms are used negatively to signal the need to control or eliminate the behavior or activity, and I believe for the most part that autistic people *need* to act the way they act. This includes talking to oneself, flapping, pacing, thumb-sucking—all the things my Nat does with autistic exuberance. I've learned from Nat and from more communicative adults with autism that it's "better flappy than unhappy."

Day habilitation, day programs, and sheltered workshops defined

Because the thrust of my book is about creating a fulfilling life in the face of a challenging disability and limited adult services, I devote a good deal of space to housing and daytime pursuits. I found that many interviewees were passionate in their discussion of traditional group homes and day programs, particularly day habilitation (also called day hab) and sheltered workshops. **Day habilitation** is defined by the federal Center for Medicaid and Medicare Services as the "provision of regularly scheduled activities in a non-residential setting, separate from the participant's private residence or other residential living arrangement, such as assistance with acquisition, retention, or improvement in self-help, socialization, and adaptive skills that enhance social development and develop skills in performing activities of daily living and community living." In day habilitation, typically, the clients are organized into large groups, with few staff to help them, and they work on social, physical, money, or daily living skills. But the staff is not trained like the teachers and specialists in public school, and so the quality of learning is often poor. Sometimes people color, watch television, or go on a walk in a mall—hardly the way to progress in a meaningful way. I prefer Nat to work, which is organized through his day program, not at his day hab center. **Day programs,** on the other hand, are often set up with more enriching activities, structure, and community-based occupations than day habilitation. Day programs can include paid work as well as trips and physical activity—they have a lot of structure, which is often necessary for people with autism, who have trouble connecting the dots of the world. Day habilitations, because they are required to be therapeutic—a medical model—are far more limited in their offerings, including that they cannot offer paid employment or education.

A **sheltered workshop** is defined by the Social Security Administration as "a private nonprofit, state, or local government institution that provides employment opportunities for individuals who are developmentally, physically, or mentally impaired, to prepare for gainful work in the general economy. These services may include physical rehabilitation, training in basic work and life skills (e.g., how to apply for a job, attendance, personal grooming, and handling money), training on specific job skills, and providing work experience in the workshop." Historically, sheltered workshops have operated within day program centers, away from the mainstream community, giving them an institutional character, rather than an inclusive, normative one. Also, sheltered workshop participants have often been paid sub-minimum wage for their work, or not at all, raising the question of the ethical and legal treatment of people with disabilities.

Many in the disability community dread *any* setting—whether day program or residence—that has an institutional feel, for fear of returning to those days of the large, impersonal, often abusive warehouses for the disabled. The history of disability rights is saddled with the ugly reality of abuse, isolation, and marginalization of its people. The documented abuse that inmates suffered is the stuff of horror films. In the 1970s, journalist Geraldo Rivera brought national media attention to one particular institution's (Willowbrook) crimes against its inmates, beginning the demand to shut them down.

And so advocates now want to be sure to avoid this possibility. However, there will always be a few residents or families who believe that the institution they have lived or worked in for decades is the best place for them. This is a minority opinion, yet it is important to consider in this era of self-determination. If indeed the trend in this country is to allow the disabled individual to determine what is best for him or her, what happens when he—or his guardians who speak for him—wants a program that is considered "institutional," i.e., a relic of the past? These are questions that are being discussed right now across the United States, in public community hearings held by Departments of Developmental Services. At present the debate is a heated one.

This anti-institutional mentality pervades day programs, too. Now the trend is also to close all sheltered workshops. The thinking behind this is that disabled people must be included in the community whenever possible. State and federal agencies, as well as self-advocates, are leading the charge toward such inclusion. How can anyone argue with that? People should not be hidden away in some center somewhere doing piecework and assembling kits, often with no pay.

Yet not *all* people agree with the wholesale condemnation of this practice for the simple reason that self-determination may be at stake. Closing institutions and sheltered workshops is a great goal, but only when we are certain that the very folks using them will benefit by moving on to more community-based programs. The sticky point comes in when there are some folks who enjoy their piecework employment at sheltered workshops.

My viewpoint is that we need to consider as much as possible the wishes of the individual. We need to be careful not to once again herd everyone into the same kind of setting—in the present, the popular ideal is community inclusiveness—if that setting proves difficult for the individual. And will the workforce be willing and able to accommodate people who need so many supports? As it is, even the "higher-functioning" disabled are grossly underemployed

We have to be careful that we don't make broad assumptions that we know what's good for another human being. We have to make room for individual preferences and skill levels. Advocates must, to the best of their abilities, assess whether the sheltered workshop employee is enjoying himself—even if to "us" (the caregivers) the work seems beneath him. Let's not eliminate something wholesale on principle. For some people, work is work, and they are glad to have a job, any job. As one autistic friend once told me, "There is no such thing as a bad job. Only bad attitudes." (Kate Gladstone, Chapter Six, 2014)

CHAPTER ONE

POST TWENTY-TWO PLANNING

Facing Transition

Beginning to plan for Nat's adulthood

When did I start facing the truth that Nat would someday have to live without me? In some ways, I thought about it the first year he was diagnosed, when he was three. Back then, I would have imagined Nat as a quiet man, spacey, kind of lost, just an elongated version of my toddler. I couldn't imagine how adult autistics looked or acted, much less how they thought. Sometimes I got a glimpse and then that door would slam shut and I'd be left outside with little Nat, peering into the keyhole.

The first time I learned about an autistic who was not a child was in a support group. One dad there had a teenager. A teenager! What was that like? I wanted to bow down at his feet and beg him to tell me. But that dad was so burdened with his own family's problems that I barely learned anything.

Contemplating Nat's adulthood was terrifying. During his childhood, I lived in the moment—though not often in a happy frame of mind. I just grabbed hold of each part of the day and pulled myself along, like I was wrenching myself across the horizontal rungs on a jungle gym.

By the time Nat was a young teen, Ned and I had to decide what our goals should be as Nat moved toward adulthood. We found ourselves at a crossroads of pragmatics versus academics. Back then it seemed like such a huge decision, and of course it was. I always knew that I wanted Nat to be as independent as possible, but until that fateful Individualized Education Plan (IEP) meeting, where we decided firmly on giving Nat a practical skills curriculum, I had not needed to face it. And facing this question can be heartbreaking to autism parents because it can signal the end of certain dreams; it can feel like you are consigning your child to a limited life. To some families, focusing on pragmatics over academics means no college, no high-level job. Of course it need not mean this; there are plenty of colleges with adapted curricula, with support services. There are community colleges that accommodate all sorts of learning styles and goals.

But I didn't know that. Moreover, I did not like to imagine the kind of manual labor job Nat would probably get. Back then, I was ashamed, because it was not the type of employment people in my family had. I look back and I understand my discomfort, but I don't feel that way now. If there is one thing I've learned in the twenty-five years of being Nat's mom, it is to have compassion for my younger self.

Ned challenged me about my attitude. "What does he need social studies for," Ned had asked me back then. I wrote about how painful this was for me in the *Washington Post* in 2002, expressing the self-doubt I had back then.

Here we were, deciding his future:

At fourteen, my son has reached a major crossroads in his life— but he doesn't even know it. While other boys his age prepare for high school and ultimately college, he is now being channeled into a strictly vocational track, to a world of lowered expectations and dim hope—and is losing his academics altogether.

Over the years, and especially recently, I have listened to politicians and school professionals swear that every child—even one as disabled as my son, who has autism—should be expected to rise to a certain level of academic achievement. Congress continues to debate just how much access to the curriculum children such as Nat deserve, and new federal legislation requires that school systems now push for every child (even mine) to be proficient in English and math in the coming decade. But I have yet to learn how, precisely, that will happen for him.

I do not blame the hardworking people who sit with him daily and figure out ways to reach him for deciding that there is no more use in teaching him social studies or literature. That there is no option for him other than skill-building is not their fault. And in our previous team meetings, the school staff made efforts to offer the state curriculum strands to my son at his level. The language around the table had always been peppered with such familiar terms as "multiplication" and "science." And even though his program was institutional in so many ways—no art on the walls, no performances, sports, enrichment, or even socialization among the kids—there was still a modicum of school atmosphere within the classrooms themselves. The teachers attempted to keep things as normal as they could, given the circumstances of fairly severe autism, and I would derive comfort from this apparent illusion of a regular classroom experience, even when the curriculum was not very inspired.

Until now. I reviewed the proposed goals for the coming year, and I saw nothing from the past. Math had become "money skills." Science and technology had become "learning to e-mail." Literature had disappeared. I asked about the state standards and how he was going to achieve them, and the room got very quiet.

I am trying to understand how in this culture of high achievement for all, this has happened. And I know, in my heart of hearts, that with all the progress made by educators and lawmakers, it is because there is still very little future for a child such as mine, just as there is so very little understood about how to educate him. We no longer institutionalize, we include. But do we really? How can we, if we still do not know how best to reach people like him? Our approaches are still in the Dark Ages, while the numbers of children out there in need are huge. These children with full-blown autism are perhaps society's greatest challenge, and yet we know so little about what to do for them. At fourteen this son of mine still sucks his thumb in public. He unabashedly loves Disney. He still has difficulty answering simple questions accurately. I understand how limited he appears to others.

It's just that to me there is so much more. I look at him and I see a quiet but passionate boy with a mischievous streak. A long-limbed kid who is a natural athlete. A person with hobbies, likes and dislikes. If I allow his educational team to decide on this strictly vocational, non-academic direction to his education, am I, too, shortchanging him? Am I asking the impossible of his school, or should I indeed be pushing the people there to work even harder for him? Should I fight to keep the academics in his life, or would I be putting pressure on him to be something he simply cannot be? Having to make this choice for him opens up wounds in my heart that I had thought long healed.

I suppose, then, that this crossroad is mine as well as his. I am being asked to bear a greater sorrow than I imagined possible, perhaps worse than the day I first learned of his diagnosis. I am to accept that this very narrow future, this nearly closed door, is the only remaining place for my firstborn son. Perhaps I should take comfort, for once, in the fact that he is not aware of what people are saying around him and about him. I guess the only thing I can do is take his hand and we will cross, together.

And so we crossed over. And it ended up being the best thing for Nat, because he learned important work skills and gained great independent-living competence. I began to feel certain in the course chosen, to truly accept that indeed Nat did not need

social studies and literature. He was a different kind of person—
not lesser, just different from the typical high school student. He
would continue to need intensive education to become as capable
as possible as a grown man.

My attention began to turn toward the adult world. At some
point in his mid teens I awoke fully to the understanding that the
more independent he could become, the better. The best thing I
could for Nat as his mother was to help him fly, as unfettered by
his disability as possible.

The first clear memory I have of actually working on Nat's
adulthood was probably toward the end of 2007, when he was
seventeen. I was sitting inside a stream of weak sunlight, in the
playroom where I keep all my files. The usual dust powdered
the reddish-brown floorboards and the windowsills. Folders
were spread out on my lap and on the gold carpet under my
folded knees. I was looking through papers—reports and dog-
eared, hastily scribbled notes I'd taken at some seminar or other
for parents. Brochures spilled out, unopened, glossy, packed
with jargoned paragraphs intended to give me hope. The letters were small and black, and they didn't really say anything.
"We're here for you." Or, "We've provided services for people
with intellectual disabilities and their families for decades." Or,
"Our adult residences offer professional, loving care for your
loved one."

I was searching for a list, a phone number. My fingers shuf-
fled through the papers like little Flintstone feet, trying to get
that big stone car moving. I felt inexplicably tired. That guy . . .
that person who'd called me a year or so back, about Nat's respite
funding, from the Department of Mental Retardation, as it was
called then. What was his name? David something? I closed the
folder and sat back on the rug and sighed.

Okay, don't just give up now; you have to do this, I told
myself. So where do I begin?

The school hadn't told me anything about whom to call,
what to see. Okay, I thought. *What am I looking for in terms of*

Nat's future? It can't be that complicated, can it? He will need to live somewhere. Who helps with that? How do you get the money for it? Agencies, vendors. Which is which? My heart was speeding up again. Deep breath.

Okay. The phone book. The blue government pages. I hefted the White Pages from its dusty shelf onto my lap and found the listings, the blue pages. A memory flickered: the government departments were called *agencies*. Our agency was the Department of Developmental Services, DDS (formerly the Department of Mental Retardation, DMR). The *vendors* were the people who provided the actual services used—such as job coaches, transportation to the workplace from the day program, feeding and toileting assistance. Vendors are mostly private nonprofits that specialize in disability services. I breathed a sigh of relief, having solved one tiny piece of the impossible puzzle ahead of me. I found some phone numbers. I called the DDS and I talked to a woman about what I was looking for: "Well, my son is seventeen, he's still in school, but I know I'm supposed to start planning for where he'll live after he is done with school, so I'm calling to find out what I should do next."

There was a pause. I think the woman actually chuckled. "He's only seventeen? Oh, you have time." I could feel her attention receding from me. *Wait! Come back! What should I do? Isn't there something I'm supposed to do* now?

But she was not interested in my son or me. We exchanged one or two more pleasantries and I hung up and put the folders away for the right time. But I knew, in my heavy heart, that she was wrong. The time was now.

The horrible familiar feeling started trickling in: helplessness mixed with dread. I was not used to feeling helpless about Nat, not anymore. It had been almost fifteen years since his first IEP meeting when I barely even understood what autism meant. And fifteen years is like sixty-five in autism parent years. A wise old bird; that was me. An owl, almost past her prime, or a leathery old hawk, seasoned from brilliant bloody kills made as a young bird. I'd had to be that way. It was a different era back then, and if you were one of the rare parents whose child had autism, there was little to no information for you, and few autism programs in the schools. Nat's early childhood had also been a world with no Internet, no one in eighty-eight, no puzzle piece ribbon. No clue.

We did in fact choose the vocational, pragmatic school path for Nat, at thirteen. Nat had been in private, out-of-district special education programs from the time he was three, so it was a natural choice for us to continue to send him to schools outside of the public schools in our town—though they funded Nat's education as required by federal law.

By fifteen he was working within his school, performing office tasks, delivering messages from the main office to personnel, even entering data and stocking shelves in the mock school store. Unlike typical high schools, who may do out-of-district placements in vocational schools for those not going on to college or who may have a few in-house vocational education opportunities, Nat's school is in fact considered a vocational school for students with autism, and so they have many contacts in the greater community, making it possible for many of their students to get real jobs. And so at sixteen his team decided to start him working in the community—at Papa Gino's, a local pizza chain, making boxes. He also began serving lunch in the school cafeteria, and cleaning the lunchroom.

In spite of all of his work experience, by the time Nat was nineteen, my anxiety had turned blade-sharp; I needed to start carving out a real future for him. Only this time, there was some movement from others around me, like stray bits of sand lifting with the breeze from the street, blowing in small circles and then softly outward.

At Nat's IEP meeting, Francie, our DDS Transition Liaison, started to get serious. Francie asked how many hours in a row Nat was capable of working, and the school people answered that he worked a few hours at each of many different jobs: making boxes at Papa Gino's, cleaning the cafeteria before and after lunch, serving lunches, and delivering coupons in the neighborhoods.

Francie asked us how many hours of work Nat clocked in each day.

The team leader, Cheryl, said, "Well, the way we do it here is he goes for two hour shifts at his various jobs."

Francie surprised us. "Not good enough," she said. "He needs to be able to work as many hours as possible in a row in order to demonstrate that he is capable of holding down a job. Can't you keep him at Papa Gino's longer, have him do both the boxes and the coupon delivery on the same days, one after the other?"

The school team members looked at each other and there was kind of a group shrug. A little flicker of irritation shot through me as I wondered if there was some silly dogmatic policy that would prevent them from making this change—Nat's school was a very bureaucratic, rigid place. They prided themselves on their consistent approach, their adherence to taking data, the quantified autistic life that leads to a productive if somewhat rote life. I'd had my fill of that unwavering attitude by the time Nat was in his late teens, but this private school had been our only option. So we were stuck with his private school program, warts and all. In the end the team was able to work out the details of a prolonged workday for Nat, however, and I was tremendously pleased.

We learned that our next step in Nat's transition out of high school was to make an appointment with our DDS eligibility office. We did not yet know if Nat was eligible for financial assistance for things such as housing, housing staff, and job coach, but we had to do everything we could to pile up reasons why he would need a lot of support as an adult. It would help, we were told, that he had been living at the school residences for the last year, and that our youngest had been diagnosed with PTSD due in part to Nat's occasional outbursts of aggression. It would matter, but it didn't guarantee anything. All I knew was that if Nat had to come home to live with us after he graduated, it would be very hard for our family. As horrible as this felt to say, I would feel like a prisoner. I loved Nat so much that my heart sometimes felt bruised and tender just looking at him and his innocence, his unknowing neediness. But I also knew this terrible truth: my own consciousness would forever be split between my own life and my life with Nat if he came home to live with us. My mind would never settle. If Nat lived with us full time, I would never be able to leave my house without arranging for someone to look after Nat, without worrying that if I didn't come back when he expected there would be trouble, and someone I care about would have to pay for it. I knew that if he did not have his own place to live, and he had to live here, that even with supports there would be times when he would be so anxious that we'd feel helpless and scared. I knew, because we had lived through that just the year before. I remembered holding his bedroom door closed while he screamed and jumped, shaking the chandelier in the hallway. One part of me was worried about neighbors calling the cops, and my other two sons' feelings of being in danger, while the other part felt Nat's pain as my own—pain from not being able to help him, merely contain him.

I went back to my files in the playroom, but this time I knew what I was looking for: any and all evaluations that talked about the severity of Nat's disability—IEPs, documentation of his violent behavior. All the way back to age three, as far as his life as an autistic person would take him.

This office of the DDS happened to be housed in the Fernald complex, which used to be an institution from 1951 to 2001 for the "severely mentally retarded." The irony was not lost on me that we were going to this same place to apply for services so that our son could live more independently as an adult—and that, furthermore, there was now a federal law changing the term "mentally retarded" to "intellectually delayed."

Soon we would be meeting with a person who would determine Nat's adult future; where he would live, and how. I was ready for a fight. I would be damned if they—I didn't really know who—would consign Nat to some hopeless life. Not after all this education. Not after how far he'd come. He was going to have a good life, and they'd have to mow me down into my grave before I allowed anything different to happen.

I came in with my head full of steam, loaded for bear with my sheaf of papers, all copied and filled out, and the administrator said, "Wow, you're hired!" I relaxed. He was actually a good guy. He gave us a great website and the name of the person in charge of our next step, which would be a discussion of services Nat required once eligibility had been determined. I started to feel a soft sweet hope in my heart.

We emerged with eligibility for a Priority One, the highest level of support needed. Even with that, we would not know the *actual* monetary sum until just a few months before he turned twenty-two. We only had the acknowledgement that Nat could potentially have housing and support staff. We did not know which sort of living arrangement would be best for Nat: a group home, or an apartment with one roommate and a caregiver.

Group home, Adult Family Care, Shared Living, and Self-Determination

A **group home** is usually run by a state-approved service provider, and is most often five people living together, with staff working on shifts. Some group homes need twenty-four-hour staffing, some even need an awake-overnight staff. Some only need staff part-time. Nat needed twenty-four-hour oversight, and this was a very expensive proposition. Indeed, it is becoming increasingly rare for states to fund fully staffed group homes, and, knowing that, I had to look into other kinds of housing solutions until we would learn exactly what Nat's funding would be.

Without understanding much about them (that would come later), I heard about **Adult Foster Care**, a Medicaid-based program that pays a caregiver a stipend to live with the person with the disability. The stipend is often less than $10,000 a year in Massachusetts, and so sometimes two disabled people with AFC funding will live together and pool their stipend money, sharing the caregiver.

A third option, **Shared Living,** offers an arrangement similar to AFC's live-in caregiver, but the state Department of Developmental Services pays the salary and the rent. We liked the Shared Living option but, not knowing what Nat's funding amount, we could not plan for that.

During Nat's nineteenth year we saw quite a bit of our DDS liaison, Francie. I grew fond of her. When she would sit across from me at our long dining room table, she seemed to really care about us. She smiled easily and her admiration for Nat shone from her grandmotherly eyes. At one of our meetings she told me about **Self-Determination**, an empowerment movement that encourages people with disabilities to exert control in their lives and to advocate on their own behalf.

She thought that Self-Determination would be a good way to go about putting together Nat's future.

Without even knowing what it was, at the mention of Self-Determination something bright pushed upward through me and opened like a flower to the sun. *Self-Determination*, I thought. *That means Nat decides. We decide.* And I knew what that meant: we would create a living situation, tailored to Nat's needs and preferences. For instance, maybe that would mean an urban lifestyle, in an apartment somewhere in Boston. He had grown up walking everywhere, taking the Boston trolleys and subway with us. Or maybe he'd live with a group of young men we would find ourselves, guys like him—active, into trips and sports.

Francie's words about Self-Determination blew across my brain and just like that, everything was clear. I was going to design Nat's adult living situation, using the models of either a group home, AFC, or Shared Living, but adapting them to exactly what Nat would need and want. I was going to control the entire process, and that was how he would have a good life. I understood this with every fiber of my being, and nothing would ever be able to shake that.

I didn't get much time to figure out how I would go about creating this good life Nat was supposed to have. Within a few weeks after she spoke those words, Francie retired. But before leaving, she made sure I had an appointment with a well-known advocate named Jeff Keilson to come over and meet Nat and discuss Nat's self-determination with us.

The morning of the appointment, I opened the door to a disheveled man with waves of white hair. His smile was open and friendly—it felt like I'd known him for a while. I relaxed a little and offered him coffee. He had a New York accent, which also made me feel comfortable because he sounded like people in my family. I had made coffee ahead of time and I was about to serve it when he asked for the bathroom. His phone rang while he was in there but instead of ignoring it like most people he answered it while he was washing his hands. This, I discovered, is Jeff, in a nutshell—always trying to do a million things at once, always anxious to help. If we could all find our own Jeff, the world would be a much better place.

We talked a little about what I pictured for Nat's future. I told him what I'd been thinking for some time now, about my ideas that were based only on what I knew about Nat, what I thought he would like, and not on any specific knowledge of the system or of existing programs. This was my vision only. I told Jeff something like this: "I want Nat to live near me. I want to be able to run into Nat or at least meet him places or know where he is on a given afternoon. He should be able to have the kind of activities he has in the community now: walk to an ice cream store, a Starbucks, the YMCA, or to be able to take public transportation. These opportunities would give Nat a sense of familiarity and as we know with autism—or at least with Nat—familiarity breeds comfort breeds happiness." I had this picture of adult Nat living in the hip big city (just like my middle son Max, at NYU), and for once in Nat's life I felt like I was going to be able to brag.

Of course, my attitude wasn't quite what it should have been, because Nat's adult life was not about my pride, my ability to crow to my friends. But these uglier emotions are part of reality, too. My love for Nat is complicated, knotted, and old, like an ancient tree. My hopes for Nat's adult life were simple, though. They centered on two things: Nat was very able to work and live with other people. Could I possibly get him this, my dream of a city apartment for Nat, with some great person looking after him, helping him become as independent as possible?

Jeff did not say yes or no. He urged me to dream, to envision it all, to come up with my picture for Nat's life and then see how to put it together. There would be parts we could do, and parts we could not do. There'd be things that fell apart, things we'd scrap, and others we would keep. We did not know how things would turn out, but we should not view any decision as a permanent one for the rest of Nat's life, anyway.

The meeting with Jeff just lit up my brain. My heart brimmed full of possibility, something I never thought I'd feel about Nat's transition to adulthood. But we were still at the beginning of Nat's journey. After that galvanizing meeting, I would often meet Jeff for coffee at Starbucks during Nat's transition days. He'd go get a napkin and scribble things on it like how the funding works in Massachusetts, and how this or that adult program works. He would listen, smiling, while I railed about the state bureaucracy that could not get off its ass and tell us what his funding would be. How could families plan at all if they didn't know if they were going to have any funding for their kid's adulthood? No wonder we autism parents are all filled with despair. Our personal finances are limited and we don't know about our child's funding until he's almost twenty-two. I didn't know what Nat would get from the government other than his Supplemental Security Income check, a federal Social Security program that is usually around seven hundred dollars a month for someone as cognitively and functionally disabled as Nat. This certainly was not enough to cover rent in Boston. Not unless I tried to find him housing in a project.

I'd huff and puff at Jeff, sitting in Starbucks with his hot water and lemon (he rarely bought anything, but I do remember him once asking the barista if he could buy just a half of a cookie). Couldn't I just have this one thing for Nat, my cool young man living in a dumpy first apartment in the city with another guy and someone looking after them? I wanted it so badly I could not stop looking at real estate ads for cheap three-bedroom apartments, and driving around cute Boston neighborhoods, and eyeing people I knew. (Nat's teachers or other aide-types or chaperones on his social group trips) as potential caregivers.

By this time, we were getting closer and closer to twenty-two, when Nat would graduate school—federal law allows someone with his degree of disability an extra four years of school, receiving services and likely training for a job. But we still had no living situation for him at all. But I had ideas. Plenty of them, and they would not let me be. And that little bit of OCD would prove to be our lifeline.

Lining up the ducks before graduation

As much as I thought I had the bull by the horns now in terms of what I wanted for Nat's adulthood, I now know there are other avenues people pursue. Nat has only been a post-twenty-two adult for a few years, and I have only begun to get a sense of perspective in how to "do" autism adulthood. As in every other phase of Nat's life, I went from feeling in the dark and alone, to getting my sea legs and plunging in and going to conferences, to sitting down with other parents to learn from them.

Chapter Two

IF YOU WANT SOMETHING BETTER, CREATE IT!

Employment and Job Training

"Start work skills at age twelve. Run the church webpage; work in a farmer's market. Let's not get trapped in the autism silo. It's a big spectrum. What would have happened to Einstein and Jobs if they'd had the autism label?"

—Dr. Temple Grandin, November 2013

Nat's early days of employment

Nat has been employed since he was fourteen—from delivering messages within his school, to wiping down tables or serving meals in the school cafeteria, to shelving items at a convenience store. I never *had* to try to find him employment. His school—a private program for students with autism—and then his day program did that for him, using their own connections in the community. But when Nat was still a teen, even though he was working at a pizza chain making boxes, I wanted more for him. My fantasy was that he would work in our hometown. For me, it was always about his hometown. I am and have always been a firm believer in community inclusion for Nat. I want him to have neighbors, people in town who know him.

Looking at his skills and his personality, I determined that our public library would be the place for him—putting stuff away in a quiet place. It made perfect sense to me. I contacted a person I knew who was a trustee at the library and told her what I was looking for. She thought it was a good idea, but somewhere along the way, amid buried emails, nothing happened. I was supposed to go in with Nat to meet her but back then I was still afraid of Nat's unpredictable behavior. He was given to biting his arm if he was frustrated, and frustration came quite easily to him. His communication skills were not developed enough for him to articulate the need for help.

It is very easy to become discouraged when you're the parent of a severely impacted autistic child. You think about all the ways things could go wrong. But we really need to fight those tendencies and plow through. Perhaps I could have made lists of my tasks and given myself deadlines for each one. Looking back, I think I was reluctant to ask the library for some support structure for Nat—an aide or some other library employee watching over him. Right or wrong, I assumed the library would say they couldn't do that. I was also concerned that Nat was far more disabled than they could handle. Nat was used to his private program where the staff was trained in behavioral techniques, where they could respond to his frustrations and outbursts in such a way that did not reinforce his inappropriate actions. I also did not think his school would send someone to be his job coach; it was impractical because his school was about twenty-five minutes from our town library. And I did not believe our own school system would find someone qualified to do the job either. Nat was out of the system—out of sight, out of mind.

My image of Nat quietly studying book spines and alphabetizing disintegrated into dust. So I let it drop, believing that his existing program would make something else happen for him. The compromise was that it would be thirty minutes away, in their town and not ours.

Planning Nat's post-graduate days — finding a day program

About a year before Nat was to graduate, I started researching day programs and day habs in earnest—obsessively, really. Funding for **day hab**, or **day habilitation**, is dictated by Medicaid, and must follow a "therapeutic" model rather than an employment model.

Day programs or **community-based day services** are provided by state-approved organizations (service providers) for people with autism. Day programs must be provided in the community and may not be in an institutional setting or a setting that has the qualities of an institution. Some day program services include job coaching (assistance on the job) and other on- or off-site work or community activities. Day programs have more flexibility in activities and offerings than day habs.

One reason I pushed for a day program for Nat was that I wanted him to have the best job possible, and in adulthood, it is the day program that does the job placement. Day habs operate under different rules and do not offer income opportunities. The other reason was that I wanted Nat's transition out of school to be as seamless as possible. To me that meant he would go right into the program from the hours of nine to three, and perhaps feel that the routine of adulthood was not all that different from what he'd known in school. But even though I was determined to make Nat's transition smooth, it felt like mine was going to be bloody. I was not ready to think of Nat as an adult. I was so afraid to go to those programs for adults and see the other disabled people he'd be with. Would I find a bunch of lost souls shuffling around from van to mall every day?

I didn't fully recognize how much disability shame I carried around in those days. The shame and the defeatism overwhelmed me so often, I wonder sometimes how I ever managed to accomplish my goals for Nat.

Some of this distress loosened up for me from a chance meeting with a colleague one morning on my commute to work. A few months into my day program research, I was riding the subway into Boston, to my job at Suffolk University, when I ran into a fellow professor from the English department. Eventually our conversation turned to what we do in our personal lives.

Often back then I didn't want to talk about Nat—my feelings, my discoveries, my heart's most important thoughts—to someone I didn't know very well. I didn't want to hear them say something ignorant about autism; I didn't want to have to educate them; I didn't want awkwardness. I wanted, rather, to choose my mode of disclosure—writing or giving talks. I felt that the general public needed to know about Nat and others like him; people need to get pushed out of their comfort zone and understand about others in society, the way I have learned from him and his autism. In doing so, I often had to push myself out of my own comfort zone and take risks, but I usually did that in a more public forum.

But there was something about this colleague's eyes that were kind; there was an ease I felt standing next to him that made me feel like I could share Nat with him. I soon found myself telling him about Nat's jobs in school. I braced myself, ready for him to react with unwanted sympathy. "Well, Nat delivers messages within his school, and he serves lunch, and he fills snack orders from other classrooms," I began.

But I was reluctant to talk about his other job, how he made boxes at Papa Gino's because that sounded like a menial job, not the kind of job I once envisioned for my firstborn—the grandson of Harvard graduates, teachers, professors; son of a mathematician, blah, blah, blah.

But then I realized what I was doing. There it was, that disability baggage I carried around—that unnecessary shame. *Stop it!* I thought. *Think about Nat, bouncing around happily, declaring in his own odd way of speaking,* "You make boxes PaGinos!" *Say it loud, say it proud.*

And so I did. I closed the lid on shame. I summoned up my pride in my guy, and proclaimed: "Nat also makes boxes at Papa Gino's." I paused. "I know, you're probably getting a little depressed at this point, thinking of a twenty-one-year-old whose favorite job is making pizza boxes." This was my attempt at a stupid joke, to break the ice and help us move on from this conversation.

Then my colleague surprised me. "No, actually," he said softly, "My first job was delivering pizza, and my favorite part of the job was when there was nothing else to deliver, so we had to make boxes. I found it really comforting."

It felt like a pile of mud had slid right off of me. Suddenly I was clean, and I could breathe. I knew then that it was going to be a really good day. And more than that, I was starting to realize that what Nat could do—work out in the community—was nothing but admirable. He could hold down a job, which is a basic adult necessity and great accomplishment no matter who you are. Best of all, it was this very skill set and all the work experience that enabled Nat to do exactly what I'd hoped for: he moved seamlessly into his new adult job stocking food at a convenience store. Soon after that, the day program moved him to a job with far more responsibility and public interface: collecting shopping carts at a supermarket.

Filling Nat's week: making peace with day habilitation

Nat is in a day habilitation for part of his week, and he works at the supermarket stacking shopping carts the other days. Having

Nat in day hab was tough for me to adjust to at first, because it is far less structured and organized than school. There were two big rooms filled with mostly developmentally disabled adults. My first reaction was that the place was pure chaos. These clients were loud and no one was telling them not to be. I looked around and saw people with very crooked teeth, poorly fitting clothes. Poor people, with lousy healthcare. Was this a place where my beautiful Nat belonged? My first, uneducated—and, I confess, snobbish—reaction was a resounding "NO." Here's what I wrote in 2011 about that day:

> *As he walked into the day habilitation today for his first day, I could feel his anxiety and his excitement, perhaps, his being at loose ends. He didn't know what to do, where to sit. We were early, so they were not quite ready for him.*
>
> *He stood there, gangly in his down coat, like a big bumpy blue lollipop—it was already too warm for that—and carrying his school backpack that only had lunch in it. A lunch he'd made. I feel so proud of that and yet so sad, too, about every little thing . . . making lunch while supervised by his mom, at twenty-two; not having the right coat on; feeling awkward and new and not knowing how to say that. Someone called his name: "Nathaniel?" And he shouted,*
>
> *"Nathaniel!" As ready as a soldier, and perhaps just as nervous. Or is that me?*
>
> *Walking back to my car, feeling those stupid tears, wanting to talk to someone, opting first to talk to myself. Is it okay? It seemed a little loose and unstructured . . . better call Ned. Ned doesn't pick up. Call Jeff, my friend and guru, who has always helped me from the very beginning of Nat's transition. Get his wise, soothing perspective.*

And so I did. And I began to realize over time, in fits and starts, that these people were just that: people. In fact, most of them were happy people. A few days later I wrote:

Two clients, a young man and a young woman, got out of a van and were so excited to see me. They had that look that many have in Nat's circles: stained buckteeth, pimples, fat. But their faces lit up when they saw me—and they didn't even know who I was. They asked who I was; they shook my hand.

I realized that the noise that had bothered me so much that first day was them calling to each other and cracking jokes. Some of them guessed I was "Nat's Mom" and they were so thrilled to see a mother there—I guessed that many of the clients were living away from their parents or that it was very unusual to see parents out of context. Not bad. Not an institution. A boisterous social hall full of people I was beginning to get to know and like.

It took him years of job experience and communication development, but by the time Nat was twenty-two he was ready to work, out in the world, a part of his community. And by the time he was twenty-four, two years after starting work at the supermarket, Nat was named Employee of the Year, complete with a plaque and a picture in the newspaper. In that picture, he stands up straight, eyes wide open, with his chest puffed out, almost holding his breath in extreme self-control. This is not just a photo of Nat getting an award; this is a picture of what pride feels like to Nat.

Self-determination and being proactive

It is remarkable how things have changed in the ten years since Nat was that young teen and I dreamed of library work for him. School systems cannot afford to send kids out to private programs anymore, and they are learning that they have to develop in-house vocational training or face hordes of angry parents.

As strained as school budgets are, the federal law IDEA (Individuals with Disabilities Education Act) mandates that special needs students get services during their school years, which extend to age twenty-two in many cases, so take advantage of the system for as long as you can.

Honoring behavior can be the bridge to communication

Nothing will happen on a large scale for our guys in the world of employment until our schools commit to vocational training *and* the rest of the world is more exposed to autism. The more we become familiar with autistic behavior, autistic social preferences, sensory issues—all of the eccentricities autism brings—the better. Familiarity morphs into understanding, acceptance, compassion, and even affection.

I turned to one of the pioneers in social skill training, Dr. Lynn Kern Koegel from the Koegel Autism Center at the University of California Santa Barbara, to understand a bit about best practice in autism adulthood real-world training. For decades Lynn has been working with her husband Dr. Bob Koegel in educational strategies for school age children, and now develops strategies for employment skill-building for college students and even adults. Lynn and Bob were among the first specialists to move away from strict behavioral modification as a way of educating people with autism, to explore motivational strategies that originated with the student's own personal interests or even obsessions. Lynn said, "When we put in these motivational components, it changed everything. Now if you get them into intervention early, 90–95 percent of them learn to talk." They called their strategy Pivotal Response Therapy (PRT).

"I do a lot of consulting, but I see programs still using out-dated stuff," Lynn said. "I see people just drilling kids, which can be completely non-motivating. When you see someone who has had a huge success in life, it's because there was somebody who had really expanded on his or her interests. And kids are a lot more disruptive if we *don't* expand on their interests."

It makes sense to use what motivates a person when he or she is learning a new or difficult task. Once they become competent in the new task, Lynn's clients with autism gain respect for their own expertise, and their self-esteem blossoms, leading to confidence, and then, ultimately, to social success. Many end up finding significant others through their obsessive interests—what was originally thought to be a detriment to their development. Lynn's research and practice demonstrated definitively that when you used autistic clients' restricted interests or repetitive behaviors, it did *not* increase the behaviors after all.

> *For example, if the kid was turning the lights on and off, I might turn off the lights and say, "on," and then "on" might be their first word. If people used the restricted interests with the little kids, we would have adults with fewer significant problems because they were so motivated to talk. And once they did become motivated doing something they really liked, it became easier and more satisfying for them to talk. Also, if we took the restricted interests and turned them into clubs, they would show appropriate behavior. For example, when we develop a social club using movies—for those students who love watching movies—the kids will start engaging socially and appropriately. Often the student with autism then becomes the most valued member of the peer group in this situation because they have accumulated so much information on this favorite topic. We replicated it in middle school and high school and even with college students, and even with some of our non-college students through our state's Department of Rehabilitation.*

Lynn told me about how she witnessed a client's empathy light go on, the year her daughter was interning there at the center with Lynn. "One day my daughter noticed that one man they were working with was really into airplanes, and she told him how she was on an airplane and a goose got stuck in something, and everything started smelling and they had to do an emergency landing.

She told him she thought she was going to die and he was totally empathetic with her. 'Well,' he said, 'you never have to be afraid of that because you know, there's always more than one engine.'"

Lynn described another such occurrence when a client of hers learned awareness of others through her own previously restricted interests. "She watches movies around fifteen times, and she's really outspoken about whether children should come to the R-rated movies. One of the students said she was at a movie and people were talking, and she was so empathetic, she related it to people bringing their babies to R-rated movies. If they're able to show that empathy, even in just those areas, you have a jumping-off point. Therefore it's not a *skill* deficit; rather, it's a performance deficit." Lynn has found that performance deficits are a lot easier to work with and improve than skill deficits.

Pivotal Response Therapy has made great inroads with autistic college students at University of California Santa Barbara, where Lynn's center for autism is located. "Most of these students get to college, they have a single apartment, they stay on their computer all day long, they might miss class, risk getting on probation, but we found that when we go through these college campus clubs and find things they really like, that we can really get them socializing, and we can decrease their anxiety and depression."

In terms of employment, Lynn believes that Pivotal Response Therapy works no matter what one's cognitive level is, and this was what interested me the most, particularly what she had to say about those like Nat, with supposedly low IQs:

> *Even those with autism who have really low tested cognitive skills, if you can get them a job, get them out there, their cognitive abilities improve. Because there's so much prejudice against people with disabilities and especially people with autism, we just put these people in settings where they don't do anything all day, we're not giving them different opportunities that an individual without autism would have so we're creating this situation where*

we don't give them social opportunities, so they're getting worse and worse. Whereas if we change society and really get them out there, they would be getting better and better.

Lynn talked about one particular adult in her clinic who picks up trash. "Nicest guy. If you talk to him, he seems to have the language level of about a three-year-old. Doesn't always understand everything. But he knows every single freeway, the airlines and flight patterns of the entire world. Knows every single birthday, never forgets it. He's brilliant but so underused. We've been trying to get him a job at the bus station or train station. But it's so hard because guys like him often don't make it past the interview."

In conjunction with University of California Santa Barbara and the California Department of Rehabilitation, Lynn sees twenty-five adults at any given time to help them practice social skills. Lynn's clients practice job social skills in particular, working toward answering potential questions employers might ask and conducting mock interviews. "The whole process is geared toward employment," she said. "We videotape them with peers and try to interview them and we look at the tapes and figure out what they're doing that we can help them with. They may be asking too many questions. Or talk too much or too little, have intonation problems, honesty problems (revealing too much), or they tend to be repetitive, or even may not have good hygiene. We work to get them job-ready. At least in California, if they have significant disabilities they can get a job coach."

Lynn has found that the problems getting employment do not stem only from the autistic person's communication, social, or cognitive skills; often it is the potential employer who is the sticking point. "At UCSB I've met for over a year with this human resource guy. 'Give me ten jobs a year for my people. Any ten jobs,' I tell him. But we ran into problems with unions, and hiring practices. But then I happened to hit on some nice people in the administration who said, 'Send them over here, we'll give them jobs in IT, delivering stuff.' So we're going to start small, and if it works for them, they'll talk to other departments."

Even with all the positive research on employment and autistic people, Lynn finds the reality discouraging: "Nationwide people are still slow to hire individuals with autism." To get people employed, Lynn believes that the autism community as well as autism researchers need to change their message about autism. "There are hundreds of studies that report on everything people with ASD can't do," Lynn said with frustration in her voice. "It's actually really easy to teach them empathy, though. Our pilot data suggests that if we have a topic around their affinity, they can show empathy without treatment."

But so much has to change in society before studies like hers truly succeed. "First of all it goes back to a core problem: everyone thinks it's okay to exclude," Lynn said. Inclusion has to happen right at the beginning, the very first time kids are exposed to other kids. Real inclusion, to Lynn, is about mainstreaming, welcoming autistic kids—and it needs to start while we're very young.

A multi-organizational effort: The Teaching Hotel

One of my favorite aspects of writing this book was discovering what people create from nothing so that their adult children can work. And some of the best career-creating efforts come in a flash of inspiration. "The real story is that I came up with the idea sitting on my porch smoking cigars and drinking bourbon," Jeff H., a dad from Indiana, said to me in our phone interview. Jeff is what I call a man's man, a fierce papa bear to his son Nash (known everywhere as The Dude), a pioneer disability advocate, and a visionary—always with a twinkle in his eye. He works in high gear all the time, focused on one goal: independence and inclusion in the community for the developmentally disabled.

Jeff's motivation is his son, of course. Although Nash does not have autism—he has Down syndrome—the circumstances around intellectual disability empowerment and the lack of vocational choices or training are extremely similar. And what Jeff has been able to accomplish to improve that situation is an inspiration for anyone.

"Nash will be fourteen in February," he said, explaining his fiery sense of purpose. Even though at the time of our conversation The Dude had eight years until adulthood, Jeff knew he had a lot of work to do in preparing Nash's community. I noted that Jeff's perspective is toward changing the world, rather than changing his son—he and his wife, Jan, have done everything they can to get Nash included as a full-on member of society. I believe that this attitude, this confident assumption that the typical community can flex, accept, understand, and connect with our guys is the best strategy that self-advocates, caregivers, and parents can employ for change. Starting from a position of certainty, righteousness, and confidence can only help our cause. Brook no arguments that contain the word "can't," or that keep the bar too low. Our guys prove again and again that they can learn, grow, and work dependably and competently.

Jeff's particular project is the Teaching Hotel. Partnering with the Marriott Corporation and the Arc of Indiana, Jeff H. has built a program from the ground up, one that will be both for transition folks and for anyone who has the ability and wants to work in the hospitality industry. The program will be tuition-based, rather than government-funded. "This is a post-secondary education, not necessarily for everyone," said Jeff. "This is a prevocational education and its students will then have that support until they're 100 percent up to speed." Jeff reasons that many people with developmental disabilities need scrupulous training—better than they get in most secondary schools—and that this may ultimately cut the need to have job coaches.

"We do have some phenomenal job coaches out there," he said, "but first we need to create the job opportunities themselves. The only way is when we parents put our heads together, reach out to people who own and operate properties, and convince them to say yes."

And so he did. Not only did Jeff secure the means toward building his dream, he was determined that the program's students would receive training where their resumes would speak for themselves. Jeff hoped to thus put an end to what he calls "pity-based employment": a practice in which companies hire disabled people as a feel-good measure rather than actually understanding that these employees have specific skills that will benefit the company.

He realized early on that the disorganization of the disability community is an obstacle to employment, and also that he himself needed to become educated in disability and advocacy. "When my son was first born with Down syndrome, my only guide post was the television show *Life Goes On*. So I got involved with our local Down syndrome organization." But Jeff found himself quickly frustrated with the very narrow focus of the Down syndrome community. He recognized that the intellectual disability community in general had so much in common, and that they should band together to build political muscle—this is why I have included Jeff in this book, because his lessons apply to the autistic population as well as those with Down syndrome.

But he soon found that even the broader disability community was "always playing defense, just trying to hold on to what we have." But he likes playing offense. "With the hundreds of millions of dollars spent nationally on grants to work on employment, and all the wishes about employment, we have not moved the dial 2 percent in the last few years."

Jeff was so inflamed by the lack of progress with regard to job creation that he sought out the help of the Arc of Indiana. He teamed up with their education committee. The end result was what they called Blueprint for Change. With the Blueprint, the Arc could plan their next steps forward, while building on the programs they had. This approach allowed them to see the progress of the disability movement in an historical context.

"We might not like sheltered workshops but at the time, they were game-changing." Jeff pointed out that sheltered workshops provided the disabled with work and the pride (and sometimes wages) that comes along with that.

But what they needed now was a new game.

"I'm a business guy. So my original concept was that we were going to have to create opportunities for making money," said Jeff, thus framing the next steps inside the real business world. "The question I asked was, 'How can we take a functional business and create internships, apprenticeships, and opportunities for them [the disabled] to learn how to work within that business—and gain the skill set?'"

Jeff told me that the whole process began to become a reality when he found out there was an empty hotel in downtown Muncie. His idea was to renovate it. But the hotel got sold before Arc had a chance to buy it. "Next thing we knew, however, the city called back."

Jeff and his wife, Jan, had grown up in Muncie. He had worked hard all his life to forge a network in his city. But this connection alone was not enough. They had to keep talking to all the parties involved, beginning with the state of Indiana, and the Arc of Indiana. Jeff and his group had made the city administration so excited with their vision that the city decided to develop some empty land in partnership with them.

"We convinced Indiana that this was a good idea. We got a five-million dollar grant to get this project started; we were going after trade financing, but the banking world wanted 50 percent equity up front (which is unheard of in banking). But the city said they'd back us. We have an amazing mayor who has a grandson with autism. He wanted to float the bond for the whole amount so we can pay the debt as soon as we can." The mayor had said to Jeff H., "If it doesn't work I want the keys to the hotel so we can do something with it right away."

Jeff set up a for-profit corporation that actually owns the hotel and pays property taxes; their debt service will likely be paid off in five years. They hired a professional manager and a renowned restaurateur.

> *We planned to build a 150-bed Marriott Courtyard attached to the convention center, but it's different than the regular hotel, for inside there will be a 35,000-square-foot, full-blown training institute and educational program. When students come in, they can learn everything from housekeeping, food service, maintenance, concierge, to gift shop and security. The curriculum was created in conjunction with Marriott University, Ball State in Muncie, IBY Tech Community College, and a combination of adaptable curriculum materials from Indiana and Purdue Universities.*
>
> *When folks complete the program, they'll have the opportunity to get a job at the hotel—30 percent of the jobs will be allocated to folks with disabilities, there will be a full restaurant, bar, room service—this is the way we designed it. They'll get a certificate from Indiana Hospitality Association. There will be three possible outcomes: trainees will be able to get a job at the Hotel. Or they can go home to their community and get a job in, hospitality, the hotel world, healthcare. Or they can go into the culinary arts, or turn this training into an associate degree.*

The Arc of Indiana owns and runs the project in partnership with the city, and Jeff is now the chair of the fundraising committee and a consultant on the project. All corporations and operations are owned by the Arc of Indiana.

Jeff H.'s real goal is to challenge everyone to take the concept and figure out what other businesses could be developed for special needs people to get training and succeed. "How do we do it in manufacturing, in distribution?" Jeff H. asked. "As much as we talk to state government, if we don't convince the business owner that this is the right thing to do, we're not going to make any progress. This is my dream and my passion," Jeff H. said.

One family's research pays off: Rising Tide Car Wash

My own education in creating opportunities for employment continues to develop. Some of the projects I've learned about, such as Jeff H.'s hotel, are beyond anything I could ever do. But everyone brings their own areas of knowledge to the table. This is about what *you* might be able to do, or how you could tweak someone else's idea and make it your own. It's all about maximizing your areas of expertise in your autistic loved one's passions and talents.

Rising Tide Car Wash is a perfect example of research and skill sets structured around the ability and interests of an adult with autism. Rising Tide was lovingly brought into being by Tom D'Eri from Florida. Tom is the Chief Operating Officer of Rising Tide Car Wash, and his father John is the co-founder and CEO. Rising Tide was developed with Tom's younger autistic brother in mind.

Tom is what I'd call a "PhD level" of a disability family advocate. I have to admit I was both in awe and even a little jealous of Tom for his skill in putting Rising Tide together. Tom was motivated the same way many autism family members are: by an autistic loved one's needs, and the prospect of an empty future. Tom told me, "My brother was going to a special school in Rhode Island but he was aging out of the school system. And there didn't seem to be hope for him to get gainful employment. We figured that out early on, and wondered what we going to do."

In 2008, John, Tom's father, had the idea of starting a small business: a car wash, a deli, or a dry cleaner—something that would be profitable, or at least sustainable. Those three businesses "are the fabric of a community," Tom said. They are the kind of businesses that are always needed. They settled on a car wash.

The first thing Tom did was to figure out the challenges faced by autistic employees. He spent time at his brother's school, observing and talking to staff. Then he talked to other entrepreneurs who had started businesses employing people with autism.

Tom discovered two things. First, people with autism are indeed good at routine work, and if you structure things, they could be *superior* employees. This finding has, of course, been documented in recent articles such as the March 2014 article in the *Wall Street Journal,* "How Autism Can Help Land You a Good Job." The second important observation about autistic employment, on the other hand, was that businesses are not set up with features necessary to employ people with autism.

Like the most successful autism disability pioneers, Tom has a vision that is larger than his own family. His biggest goal is to get society to think differently about autism—to think of the autism spectrum disorder as a business *advantage,* not just something to accommodate and tolerate. He reasoned, "Like the sustainability movement in 1995, going green was not at first thought of as a business advantage. We wanted to put across the message, 'We are successful *because* we employ people with autism.'"

Tom started to connect with people in the car wash industry whom he saw as the best in the business. He went to Sonny's Enterprises in Tamarac, Florida, run by Paul Fazio. Paul was skeptical. He said, "I don't think you can do this, but we'll give you everything you need to get this done." Paul lent them his car wash, and in nine weeks over the summer, Tom recruited, trained, and employed fifteen young people with autism.

They bought their first car wash a few months later, renovated it, and employed thirty-five guys with autism; they've been operating since then. Since opening, they have quadrupled their business, and they are profitable. Using supervisors who are neurotypical, Rising Tide manages to provide great job support for the employees with autism. Tom found that they did not need to give any special autism training to the supervisors; that the supports came naturally over time because the managers got to know their employees. Tom told me that he is, however, currently working on a "'management guide' for coaching and leading people with autism. It seems to be a helpful resource to draw on when they are working through an issue with an employee, and for new managers to feel more comfortable in their roles."

Tom and his father did hit a snag when it came to paying for their operation. Banks were not willing to risk such an unproven investment. They had to invest an enormous amount of their own money to get a prototype to see if the concept even worked ($75,000). Then they had to invest about two million dollars to open the car wash to the public. "We've now recovered one million dollars through a mortgage and the other one million should be fully returned by the end of the third year of operation. On our second location, we've received SBA financing through Paradise Bank for 80 percent of the project cost." Now that they have had so much success, a bona fide, profitable business model, Tom and John say that for others starting a car wash like Rising Tide, it would not be nearly as costly, and banks would be willing to underwrite them. Tom said he would even be willing to help other parents start up the business and manage the site. Working with a day habilitation was also an option in Tom's view—and what an unusual and productive day habilitation that would be. Tom said, "We're currently working to fundraise for Rising Tide University, which will provide training and support services for those interested in copying our model." The fact that Rising Tide turned a profit in its first year is not only a testament to Tom and John's skill; it proves that the right kind of jobs and supports is pretty much all it takes to get people with autism to thrive at work.

"We're trying to create a business built for people with autism that is also valuable to the community. Our employees are very rarely late, and they follow our processes to the record." (Why am I not surprised? That good ol' ASD stereotype of sticking to routines doesn't come from nowhere.) Tom pointed out that countless families across America own a small business. He felt that they, too, could probably employ their loved one. In the end, it may be as straightforward as that for families like the D'Eris—and mine.

We have to take things into our own hands rather than wait for opportunities to come along. Like Tom and his father, we parents have to be fearless in trying, and have faith that our autistic loved ones can do it, provided that the tasks make sense for their personalities and skills. If parents or caregivers start to analyze their autistic family member's talents, hobbies, even obsessions, and continue to think about what is right there in the community—a library, a supermarket, a car wash—then isn't it possible for us to prove to the rest of the world that our children are a wealth of untapped potential? As Dr. Lynn Kern Koegel would say, we start doing this when our children are young when we bend over backward to find something they can play with appropriately, or some pursuit in common with other peers.

When Nat was about ten, for example, he was enchanted by photos of places he'd visited. He would spend long periods of time staring at pictures on the computer, flipping through them over and over again with the force of obsessive-compulsive behavior. But Ned figured, why not harness that passion and channel it into play? So Ned designed a way to string together photos of favorite routes and destinations using software he'd created (this was in 2001, before links were commonplace), and he came up with "Nat's World," a video game where Nat could click to his favorite spot. There is no difference in coming up with work solutions for our adult autistic children.

A cottage industry born from Legos: Made by Brad

Sometimes true inspiration is born of the deepest despair. Mark, an autism dad from Alberta, Canada, could not bear for his dear son Brad to founder in adulthood. Brad had too much potential for that. But with few supports or financial resources, as well as living through some very dark times, Mark was at a loss for a while as to what Brad could do with his life.

But Mark dug deep into his knowledge of his son, and found that through Brad's lifelong love of Legos, he could come up with a business for him. Although Mark had a completely different way of doing things for his son Brad than car wash kings Tom and John, there are some very stark similarities—namely relentless determination. For example, Mark told me that throughout Brad's life, his reaction to autism was, "We're going to beat this thing."

We are all human, however, and we all hit bottom, so we have to give ourselves the time to recover. And indeed, by the time Brad was fifteen years old, Mark had run out of solutions—and energy. Like so many autism parents, Mark hit the lowest point when his son was a teenager. Mark and his wife were moving to the city and they decided that it was time for Brad to move to a group home, which also proved difficult. "The night before dropping him off at the group home, we had to stay with him at a motel in the city. He didn't think we belonged in that hotel so he took our luggage and threw it off the balcony where our car was parked below. I made him pick it up. The cycle went on all night. I just didn't know what to do. I knew we had to stay there for the night. I didn't know if I should call the ambulance, the police or what. It confirmed for me that I had reached my end."

Eventually both Brad and his parents adjusted to the new situation. Brad got used to the group home after a while, but Mark knew that if Brad only had the group home in his life, he would have nothing purposeful to do. After he graduated, at twenty, Brad had absolutely nothing in his life. "The year he turned twenty I call his 'Year of Sadness,'" said Mark. "It's impossible to expect staff to invent and carry out a program. They will concentrate on delivering the domestic things, day-to-day tasks."

Mark fully understood the realities of limited staff in group homes. I have found this is true in terms of most direct care workers. As well-intentioned and loving as they may be, they neither have enough training nor earn enough money to allow them to go beyond activities of daily living tasks with their autistic clients. This is not an indictment of the employees, but rather a fact to be noted by the family going into autism adulthood. Until the adult services system can do more in terms of funding and training, families must be as creative and proactive as they can be for their children. Once you accept this fact, you can move on to action, just as you did when your child was first diagnosed.

Mark knew that it was out of the question for Brad's residential support staff to help him with a job. He realized that improving Brad's life was, in the end, up to him. Necessity is the mother of invention, and so began an Ikea-furniture assembly business for Brad. "When he was young, he built models; he got better and better, and then we brought Lego into the scene. I schemed up a way to have a guy hired to work with him at his school; the end result was that I was able to direct the program at school, and he was able to build some really big Lego projects—up to one thousand pieces." Mark always made sure Brad was building something different to challenge him to solve new problems. He felt this was good therapy for his son. In this way, Brad learned how to follow directions, which would turn out to be an excellent basis for the furniture assembly business.

Once Mark had the idea of having his son become a freelance furniture assembler, he made a promotional video for Brad, and then they promoted it on the Internet. It turned out to be an "overly successful promotion," Mark said, a soft wonder in his voice. "We were trying to get some jobs from the local area. The video spread all over the world. It was quite pleasant that so many people were interested."

Mark, like all of us, lives with a lot of uncertainty about what more to do for his son. For all of us, as Mark said, our children are a work in progress. But for Brad, this small business venture seems to be working. Not only does the assembly of the parts feel natural and easy to him, but Mark also feels that Brad's job, which is five days a week, is one big key to his newfound confidence and peace. Brad goes into people's homes and gets to be the leader in the situation. He has to assess the situation and figure out what to do. This enterprise has been successful because Mark and his wife have matched Brad's skills and hobbies with gainful employment.

And Brad's parents are not finished with Brad by any means. There's no rest for the autism parent who must constantly watch and analyze their adult child and decide if the current situation is still satisfying and worthwhile. Mark may soon decide to focus on other aspects of Brad's life. "Might go down to three days a week. Skating, bowling, we want him to do those kinds of activities. We want him to keep up his education, to use an iPad—he can print, he can type, but he actually does not recognize the words yet. He uses sign language by making a single sign, not a sentence. I'd like him to be communicating," he told me.

Creating an opportunity in your community

Autism families look to each other to learn what they need to know. It starts with the first days of diagnosis, and strengthens through support groups, the Internet autism community, and organizations that are everywhere, like Special Olympics. Our own town has a strong Special Olympics program that Nat has been part of for over ten years, which is one important way that he has been able to remain connected to his hometown. He has grown up with a handful of developmentally delayed teens and adults. While our children practice and compete, we parents naturally start talking on the sidelines and by now are good friends.

Lately, some of the families have begun to meet regularly to learn from each other about employment and housing. Because of all my research for this project, and also because Nat is a little bit older than the other kids, I have spoken to the group in the past about housing options. In addition, two of the fathers in the group have done a great deal of research around employment possibilities. The parents are very interested in starting a non-profit that would run a small business—such as a hydroponics nursery or a bakery. We have communicated with other parents who have already succeeded in adventures like these, or who have expertise that could help. It is likely that in the near future, we will each have to kick in some seed money and/or do our best to fundraise in order to begin a 501(c)(3) nonprofit. This won't be easy; each parent in the group works full time and has many responsibilities, but we have all found that we need to take the initiative ourselves in order to ensure our child's future. I am looking forward to this next phase in our and Nat's life, where he might be able to work alongside lifelong friends, in our town, where he will be overseen by his community and not strangers. And so, even though I am happy with Nat's supermarket work and those who supervise him, I still have dreams for him that I will continue to pursue.

Autism parents have to keep moving, exercising great diligence. We don't get to rest on our laurels. We want to see our children at their best. We are the first ones in their lives who see their potential, who feel their greatness, and who believe in our kids more than any others do. What we have to realize is that sometimes the answer is right there, within the child. Parents need not undergo training and study the intricacies of the state system, but you should be your child's most powerful advocate. You don't have to buy and create an entire operation like Tom and his father did, but you can take a page from their book and cannily assess what's out there, what services a community relies upon, and how your child fits into that. Capitalizing on autism's demand for routine and structure, you can perhaps fit your autistic adult family member into a business that demands just that. Sometimes you can simply look at your child, like Mark and his wife have done, and figure out what he can do. I believe that is what all successful autism parents do. That is the keystone for building our child's connection to his community.

Disability-Based Day Options Resources

- Among some of the helpful and relevant options offered by Ocali are listings such as funding sources for employment as well as activities and interventions to help with successful employment: www.ocali.org/project/tg_employment
- Arthur and Friends Hydroponics has a template for small agri-businesses to employ mostly people with intellectual disabilities: www.arthurandfriends.org
- Rising Tide Car Wash: www.risingtidecarwash.com
- The Teaching Hotel information is listed on the Arc of Indiana website: www.arcind.org/training-institute
- Check out Roses for Autism, a florist company in Connecticut that has created an easily replicated business that employs autistic people: www.rosesforautism.com
- Lee and Marie's Cakery is a small community-based New Jersey bakery business offering a template for others to create for people on the autism spectrum: www.leeandmaries.com
- Stuttering King Bakery is an Arizona baked goods business started by Matt Cottle, an autistic young man, and his mom—the name was inspired by the film *The King's Speech* and the challenges King George VI had with his verbal disability: www.stutteringkingbakery.com
- Autism Speaks is wisely moving its efforts into the autism adult world; one of their first initiatives is their Employment Toolkit, designed to help those with autism navigate the working world: www.autismspeaks.org/family-services/tool-kits/employment
- Agricultural Communities for Adults with Autism: http://ac-aa.org has a comprehensive list of farmstead options.
- Remember: college should be a viable option for many young autistic adults. The Autistic Self-Advocacy Network

(ASAN) offers a helpful resource written by autistic people about their own insights into coping with college: www. autisticadvocacy.org/projects/books/navigating-college
- Also helpful for college information and autism, the organization College Steps provides curricula to colleges and universities to accommodate all learning abilities. College Steps showcases what some institutes of higher learning have been able to do for their disabled students: www.collegesteps.org
- A terrific resource is the Arc of the US's Autism Now initiative. See their website for a thorough explanation of Medicaid and job supports: autismnow.org/on-the-job
- The Department of Labor has a Workforce Recruitment Program for College Students with Disabilities, which is "a recruitment and referral program that connects federal and private sector employers nationwide with highly motivated . . . recent graduates with disabilities who are eager to prove their abilities in the workplace through summer or permanent jobs": www.dol.gov/odep/wrp
- For a state-by-state breakdown of programs, see www.medicaidwaiver.org
- See the National Adult Day Services Association for more information on day programs and providers: www.nadsa.org
- Do2Learn is a job training and social skill site jammed with tips and resources: www.do2learn.com/JobTIPS
- According to their website, AbleLink Technologies offers "cognitive support" help through "picture-and-audio based Apps for the iPad, iPhone, and iPod Touch": www.ablelinktech.com/index.php?id=24
- Attainment Company offers an abundance of assistive technology: http://www.attainmentcompany.com/assistive-technology
- The Fraser website describes the app QuickCues as being "designed for iPods and iPhones that helps teens and young adults on the autism spectrum handle new situations and

learn new skills": www.fraser.org/Resources/Products/
QuickCues.aspx

Note: Many thanks to one of my younger and very successful autistic friends, Chloe, who has benefited from all of the
above.

Books

- Ron Suskind's book *Life, Animated: A Story of Heroes,
  Sidekicks, and Autism* is about affinity therapy, and how he
  figured out how to create a meaningful day for his autistic
  son, who draws expert Disney cartoons: www.ronsuskind.
  com/books/life-animated
- *Developing Talents*, by Dr. Temple Grandin and Kate Duffy,
  gives advice and strategies for people on the autism spectrum (Autism Asperger Publishing Company, 2008).

Lessons Learned About Fulfilling Daytime Pursuits

- Be prepared for meeting other developmentally disabled
  adults. Try to remember that an unusual face is just that:
  an arrangement of features that you don't see every day. It
  means nothing. A voice that speaks in grunts or not at all
  is still fully human, and with an inner life.

- Start a notebook. Save business cards and telephone numbers.
- Break down your research into baby steps, but start early (way before your child turns twenty-two) so that you have the chance to do it your way. Maybe you do things in bursts, like me: one appointment or maybe ten, and then none for months. Whatever works.
- Understand the key players, the names of the state agencies, departments, and service organizations involved with day programming.
- Cultivate a positive relationship with your state agency point person (the agency might be Department of Developmental Services or it might be Vocational Rehabilitation Services). Be sure you are on their radar screen as the pain-in-the-ass parent. No one wants to be that parent, but you have to be. If you aren't assertive by nature, pretend to be: fake it till you make it. Be nice, be courteous, but be in their face.
- Go to transition workshops. Pick one transition to adulthood workshop per year so that you don't become overwhelmed. Write down your questions in your notebook. Also, see www.fredconference.org for state-of-the-art conferences on transition to adulthood.
- Find a mentor—find two, find ten—and learn everything you can from them. Then, pay it forward: become one for someone else.
- Visit day habilitations and day programs. The providers vary in quality and goals; some do highly individualized curricula and others have more of a general schedule with a choice or two. Tour it and get a good feel for it and the clients it serves. Are they engaged? Happy? What kind of job connections does the provider have within the community?

- Look for natural allies and communities, such as other parents you meet at the Special Olympics or workshops, and think of them as your potential business partners.
- Above all, give yourself a break, take your time, but still: get going.

CHAPTER THREE

HOME ISN'T
BUILT IN A DAY

"Keeping your sense of priorities is a must. Everyone needs to accept the idea that the house is going to be simple, without fancy furniture and in-ground swimming pools"

—Diane, the force behind Juniper Hill Farms in
Pennsylvania

As we edged toward Nat's adulthood, I threw myself into figuring out where he would live. In the last few years of school he had been living in the residence there—a group home in a neighborhood twenty-five minutes from our home.

For Nat's adulthood, I wanted him to live the way he always had. We live in an area of Boston with shops, restaurants, a library, coffee shops, and ice cream parlors, all within walking distance to us. My idea was that I would find an old fixer-upper house or condo, and a service-providing agency—like the one Jeff Keilson, my guru, worked for—could buy it and fix it up. I would then find a way for Nat and some roommates to pay the rent.

I went with my friend Susan, who is a realtor and neighbor, and we found a really cute three-to-four-bedroom house right nearby in a great part of my town. It was a bit run-down but it was affordable—at least what passes for affordable in my Boston suburb. Nat could have two roommates like him and a caregiver. The caregiver could live in the fourth bedroom rent-free.

I could just see the whole thing. It was perfect. I imagined painting it all of Nat's favorite colors. I imagined big loud young men stretched out in the high-ceilinged living room, rejoicing every time the T went by (the D-line ran right behind the house). Many autism families know how much our guys like trains, after all. How much better could it get? I thought of how they could go on walks with their caregiver (three young men could share one using Adult Foster Care money, if they qualified) to all Nat's familiar haunts, buying brownies at the coffee shop, candy bars at the pharmacy. It would be so easy for them to live there without even having to buy a car for the house because they could walk to the supermarket. They could join ZipCar if they needed wheels. They could use The Ride, which is run by the T for people with disabilities; it is a van that picks riders up directly from their homes and takes them to work. Even though at the time Nat was probably not quite ready for The Ride, his using it became another goal in my mind. It still is.

I was so obsessed with making this happen for Nat, I could think of nothing else. My excitement and energy felt like the way I planned before he was born. This was like awaiting the birth of baby Nat because I felt full of hope! And so at times, paradoxically, the housing process made me excited. I felt proud of understanding the system, of the helpful connections I'd made, of the vision that I had. My mind was on all its cylinders. Nat's adulthood was not making me sad or scared (at least some of the time), because I had explored every dark corner of it that I could. I felt I was leaving very little to chance or the vicissitudes of state budgets.

House chasing: exploring every option

First and foremost, I learned to get on waiting lists. But while most state governments have programs for those who qualify, the waiting lists for those benefits are often very long. So, secondly, I learned that it is a good idea to forge ahead with your own ideas while still waiting on those lists. I spent about two years learning about programs and making contacts. I had endless coffees with people in the know. I went to exhausting meetings and had jaw-grinding conversations with bureaucrats. I explored any avenue to get my house for Nat—from creating a Limited Liability Corporation (LLC) or a nonprofit and doing some fundraising event to raise money to fund a house, to buying a bedroom in a private group home, to seeking a Section 8 housing voucher, which is part of a federal program that provides affordable housing to low-income citizens.

But first, because I did not yet know if the state would fund Nat's house expenses and staff, I began with the worst possible scenario—the assumption that we would have to pull together resources and bits and pieces of funding venues on our own. I started focusing on finding other families whose sons could be Nat's roommates. Once again Jeff came through for me, with two potential young men. I met with each family and we started to meet fairly regularly to talk about what we envisioned. I told them about my dream—to have Nat live in a part of Boston near us, so he could walk to interesting shops and take public transportation. They seemed amenable to this. One red flag that popped up, but that we duly ignored, was that we three families were from different regions and so our Department of Developmental Services area directors might not all agree on letting us share our funding. The families met at Jeff's house to talk about how we envisioned the shared house.

As usual, however, I pushed a bit too hard. For one thing, Nat had already lived outside of our home, while neither of the other two young men had. Even though the families thought they were ready, they probably were not. But they could not articulate that because they didn't know it, and I grew impatient.

I ignored their concerns and dove right into finding real estate. I found an apartment that I thought was a perfect place, in a neighborhood full of college students. It was kind of a dive, but it was big enough and we could just about afford it. And actually, a dive was an appropriate living situation for a young man of Nat's age.

But when the other two families saw it, they hated it. I thought this was unfair, because they just didn't know how great a deal it was for this neighborhood in Boston. They were suburban families and did not understand what we would have to be willing to accept if we wanted our children to live in Boston. I told them this rather emphatically. Before I knew it, both families had pulled out.

I continued searching for other parents whose sons were similar to Nat in hopes of starting an LLC to buy a house together, or to rent a house and all chip in for the rent. The rent would come from 75 percent of our sons' Supplemental Security Income (SSI). That would give us about five hundred dollars each for rent, so we would all have to supplement them monthly. And this was only rent. How would we pay for a staff person?

First things first, I told myself. I worked on a mission statement and read up on how to do LLC's and nonprofits. And while meeting with these families and trying to get them to commit to my idea, I kept asking around town about any other options—perhaps a first time homeowner loan in Nat's name, and even grants.

During my quest, I stumbled upon a local organization that created private group homes—you just had to buy a bedroom in the house, as you would a condo. But I didn't want to commit funds that are as permanent as buying a room in a home that I didn't own, especially given that this would be Nat's first adult living situation. I felt that you never know what mistakes you'll make the first time around; I am the queen of trial and error—emphasis on "error." And so I was anxious about the idea of possibly having to sell his bedroom condo if the whole thing didn't work out. Still, this was an idea that I kept in the back of my mind. My goal was for him to live outside of our home, and so I had to explore every option.

My next idea was to connect with larger nonprofits known for their special needs programs, like Combined Jewish Philanthropies, to see if they would give us a grant for a down payment on a house. Or perhaps they could pay for start-up costs, too, or renovations. I actually secured the promise of a very sizable gift from them, but ultimately turned it down because it came with certain requirements we could not meet.

I realized I needed to learn more ways of affording a home for Nat, and so I sat down over coffee with a helpful administrator from CJP who knew of other ways to acquire housing. She told me about the Federal Section 8 program. Section 8 provides housing vouchers for very low-income housing—just two-thirds of one's SSI. The catch—and there's always a catch—is the decade-long waiting list. Section 8, after all, is not just for people with disabilities; all sorts of populations are eligible, such as homeless families and the elderly, as well as recovering addicts.

But I discovered a "secret": the project-based Section 8. A project-based voucher is assigned to a building rather than a person, and so it stays with the building. The project always remains subsidized, and all eligible candidates can apply for it. A project-based Section 8 tends to be easier to find than receiving the mobile (person-based) Section 8 voucher, because towns are likely to have buildings available that they want to develop.

I met with my own town's housing authority, and I learned that they were indeed looking to build a few more affordable units using project-based vouchers. The catch here was that others would apply once the project is open, and there was no guarantee Nat would get it. So even if we gathered just the right roommates *and* the right staff at the precise moment—a big if—nabbing the apartment ahead of other applicants was a roll of the dice. I was about to move ahead and solidify my group of parents anyway, but then we learned that the state had given Nat Priority One status, so he would have a place in a group home run by the state. Because of his Priority One, we would not have to find a way to pay for housing or staff. Priority One is the brass ring in adult services. The catch there is that your guy has to be severely disabled enough to qualify. I used to joke grimly, "The good news is that Nat's a Priority One. The bad news is that Nat's a Priority One."

Once we learned that Nat had his funding, we shifted our energy to finding Nat a slot in a group home. The problem with this was that I did not want Nat placed in just any group home. I wanted to have a say in what the home was like. I wanted the house to be close by. I wanted the other housemates to be of a similar age and disposition to Nat.

But could that be done? Not according to my DDS liaison. "Oh, that's not how we do it," she told me. But luckily, I knew about Self-Determination and Person-Centered-Planning, the philosophy and government policies created around enabling individuals with disabilities to live in their homes (not institutions) and participate in their communities to the fullest degree possible. And so I understood that Nat, and his family as his proxy, could design his own adulthood. Beware of bureaucrats who say "No." There may be some give there if you push back.

I said, "Well, actually, I heard that we can put a home together if we have an appropriate group of roommates for Nat." This was all it took for her to relent, though with a frown. Autistics and their family members have got to be persistent with public agencies. It's not that the agencies are evil. Their behavior toward their clients is not, for the most part, due to malice or anything mean-spirited, but rather from being burned by family-created houses that fall apart. They are constrained by budget and understaffing. Also, it costs them more to build a new home for five rather than fit the one person into an existing home.

I think of my assertiveness as a way of helping everyone concerned: if I can come up with a viable solution for Nat, then that's less work for the Department of Developmental Services. Maybe they don't like me, but that just does not matter when it comes to my son. Or yours. Again, if you get nothing else from this book, remember to become a pain in the ass! Pretend to be one if you're not. It's the only way.

Eventually I invited about ten families to my house just to put our minds together and discuss what we were each looking for. Although it was clear that we all wanted a nice group home and we all liked each other, it was not at all clear how to proceed. I could not get anyone to commit to Nat's group home because of the inconvenient fact that there was no actual house yet, but we could not have DDS fully commit to a house without a cohort of Priority One roommates.

Post twenty-two had become a huge catch-22, a vicious cycle that left all of us in limbo.

However, Jeff encouraged us to keep meeting, to solidify our group, and to do all the legwork for the state. Get our ducks in a row and then present a project to the DDS that they could not refuse. So I kept looking for an affordable house that fit all of the state's rigorous group home requirements (like a back exit for every floor, a fence protecting the housemates from the street). And, of course, the other families had to keep pressuring the DDS to commit residential funding to their sons.

The group kept getting together for barbecues and dinners, and we eventually tightened up and began to feel like an extended family. We brought our guys to the gatherings and were delighted with how they got along—in their own mostly nonverbal way.

I drafted the following statement that we could all agree on that would make us seem more serious and dependable as a group, and thereby encourage DDS to permit us to establish a group home. I believe that anybody considering setting up a home for their autistic loved one would benefit from writing down their vision to be as clear as possible with any funding agencies, and also to be sure that everyone else involved agrees on what the home would be like.

Nat's Group Home Mission

To create a small, affordable group home in Xtown, MA, a town that is already diverse and accepting of all different populations and is close to Boston and many cultural attractions and opportunities. This home would be specifically geared toward young men with moderate to severe autism.

Description of Home:

1. Number of tenants varies according to funding levels: anywhere from three to five.
   a) Three tenants and one live-in 24/7 caregiver, asleep overnight but on the same floor;
   b) Up to five tenants with rotating shifts of 24/7 staff, with ratios of: 2:5, 1-2:4, and 1:3;
   c) Caregiver would have his/her own bedroom, preferably his own bathroom, and some office space.
2. Tenants are expected to be out of the home 9-3, M-F in day programs or jobs, which would leave the caregiver free time during the day.
3. Saturdays and Sundays tenants would have staff when they are in the "program." Some (possibly all) might go to their family homes for part of the day on Saturday, Saturday night, and part of the day on Sunday.
4. Home must be close to a T line to encourage community outings and greater opportunities for socialization and entertainment. The home would ideally be first floor, to

contain noise from any excessive pacing of these tenants. Hopefully the home would be located on a side street for greater walking safety.

Even after we knew we had a bona fide group, we ran into some snags. We could not agree on a house. One mom wanted all new appliances, walls, floors, but didn't care if the house was in the middle of nowhere, while I felt the opposite. I started to gnash my teeth privately. At times I wanted to just quit the whole thing and just keep Nat home with us. Sometimes I fantasized about building an apartment in our basement and hiring a caregiver for him, rather than try to make it work with other families. I began to realize that families like mine—who are so used to fighting the system for everything their autistic kid's needs—can actually be a bit contentious with each other. I joked with Jeff and Ned frequently: "They're all nuts, like me." They would laugh, of course, but they also knew how to steer the conversation to smoother, positive waters, and help keep me sane and on track (a full-time job).

Eventually we settled on a group home in a lovely suburb of Boston, a sunny spot on a cul-de-sac with a big yard, basketball hoop, deck, patio, and grill. The situation was a bit of a new arrangement for the DDS, because one of the families actually owned the house and the DDS funds would go to the family. But the DDS agreed it was a good group of young men, with strong committed families, and a lovely house. So that spring, five months after he turned twenty-two, Nat moved into his first adult home, and we breathed a huge sigh of relief. We had done it. We could finally sit back and relax. The house was lovely, with sun pouring in most of the windows and preservation land adjacent. At first, he had just one housemate. I liked the caregiver, and I loved the staff support person, John, who had worked part-time as Nat's staff person in our home.

We set up a general schedule, which had Nat coming home on the weekends; we wanted to keep his life as similar to his school group home life as possible. My thinking was that since this wasn't a home situation with us, the model we could link it to in Nat's repertoire was the school residence. I have always found that giving Nat a point of reference solidifies his understanding of any new setup.

We had trouble almost immediately. There was friction between the other family and one of the staff. None of us had realized just how much we should have spelled out our expectations of the staff. This made for a lot of awkward phone conversations where I felt I was being put in the middle. To be fair, I was putting myself in the middle because I wanted to know everything that was going on, but in doing so I was inviting confidences that ended up destroying the group dynamic. The relationships began to deteriorate.

Another two families moved in, making it now a home of four young men—we were all friends from the autism world—and we were all trying to make it work. Any house of people is bound to encounter rough spots, and that was how we looked at it. We planned parties and picnics and felt like the arrangement was working. But the underlying fissures at the beginning were widening.

The live-in caregiver left and we found ourselves in the position of hiring a replacement, but the families could not agree on a candidate. The agency made the final decision and this angered the family that owned the house.

No one wanted it to come to this, but three of the families agreed to move out—to leave the house and the first family, the young man who had been Nat's first housemate. The remaining families now had to find a different home. The agency had a house that was not being used at the time, and it was in a sad, poor part of town forty-five minutes away. But this was to be temporary until we could find a house in Boston, which was our region.

This was a stressful, unhappy period for the parents, and likely the staff and the guys themselves, following the previous stressful unhappy period when the first home broke up. But soon we worked out a similar schedule to what we'd been following, which helped the guys adjust. And luckily we retained the staff that had been with the first home, and they were very invested in making this new situation work. They cared so much for the guys and worried about the transition. But the new house manager—again, John Excellent—painted walls bright colors and arranged the rooms with lively curtains and posters and we felt we could make a go of it. Once again the families were determined to give the home a family feel, and we planned birthday parties and holiday celebrations. John and I brought Chanukah to the house; another family provided some fun Halloween activities and treats.

About six months into it, the agency found a lovely newly built home in a suburban part of Boston, not far from where the first house had been. The house was only affordable because it was on a very busy street in an industrial area. The staff came along with us, and it was a beautiful new beginning.

During the early summer, we got to know other group homes nearby and we tried to have all those residents socialize every now and then. One such group was unofficially called the "Chinese House." This home, though funded by the state, had been organized much like ours—through the efforts of like-minded parents. In this case, the parents were Chinese-American families who wanted to maintain Chinese culture for their sons. Housing success depends on this kind of alliance: strong similar culture and values, and long-term relationships among the families. There is no guarantee, of course, but these ingredients help eliminate some potential obstacles to getting along.

Publicly funded group home with a theme

I recently learned about another such group from an old friend of mine. Robin (named changed to protect her family) and I met in a support group started by parents at our preschool when Nat was five. Robin has a son a few years younger than Nat. At the time, she had no idea what was wrong with her son, but she suspected autism.

We've both come a long way. We now meet for coffee a few times a year to catch up on the latest in the autism world. At our most recent get-together, she told me about a successful group home started by parents she knew at her son's school—where else would a great living situation develop but among parents who have bonded over autism?

What started out as a community of many families ended up as two group homes run by the Department of Developmental Services. The houses are an example of what planning and the support of a knowledgeable organization can do. The houses are the result of a partnership with the Boston Higashi School, the DDS, and a service provider—a local Arc. Though they are not free of problems—what is?—they seem to have what it takes to stay strong.

Robin told me over coffee how they did it. A few years before her son was to turn twenty-two, she looked around his school for students of similar age. Higashi is a small school with a particularly holistic philosophy of "Daily Living Therapy," which emphasizes relationships, a healthy diet, vigorous exercise, musical instruction, regular integration with the community, and high expectations of behavior. Ned and I had actually wanted Nat to go to Higashi at one point in his life, but back then he was doing well on his medications, and at that time Higashi was opposed to most medications. Their belief was that they would succeed in their training without relying on anything but natural structure and rigor. Most of the Higashi students would be considered on the severe end of the spectrum, yet they end up learning musical instruments (Higashi has a fantastic jazz band), loving outdoor exercise and sports, even riding unicycles. If I sound like an advertisement for Higashi, I'm not surprised. I'm now a member of their Advisory Board and a fan for life.

I met with Dan, a Higashi dad who had a dream of buying an unused complex in the town of Sharon, hoping to establish an entire Higashi community there, similar to what the students now had at their school. This setup would be complete with housing, recreation (there was a swimming pool), and paid work.

This kind of vision is the dream of many autism parents, who want their loved ones in a place that understands them, a place in the community yet separate in the ways that matter most: work, play, and living. The idea is that the residents there have so many things in common: most importantly, their educational training at Higashi. They could easily share staff because they share the familiar context for learning and behavior. I thought this was a wonderful no-brainer. How could anyone find a problem with a living situation like this, with so much built-in support? And, considering that the students—especially those who had lived at Higashi during the school years—had enjoyed a very similar experience prior to graduating, wouldn't this idea be a very logical next step?

The town did not see it this way. The project, ultimately, was too big for the site chosen. The Higashi parents did not give up. Instead, they adapted to the DDS strictures and tried to hold onto one of the most important pieces of their plan: the training of the staff.

While aggressively keeping in touch with her DDS area director, Robin and a few other Higashi parents started looking around for a service provider that would be willing to support Daily Living Therapy training of staff for the home. Robin's group had to jump through the usual bureaucratic hoops, but that is nothing new. My group had to do this as well, because we could not be certain that the DDS would agree to allow a house to begin with only one twenty-two year old—the others would be aging out within the coming year. This kind of arrangement is one of the reasons the DDS does not jump at the chance to start group homes from scratch, because it costs more to acquire a new home and keep it running with all the appropriate staff if there are so few funded residents to inhabit it at the beginning. Far easier to find existing slots in up and running places than to start a house that is nearly empty for a while. In Robin's case, there was also the matter of a potentially unethical situation of denying other (in this case non-Higashi) twenty-two-year-old candidates for the new house while they waited for their group to turn twenty-two.

Nevertheless, DDS tries to respect the tenets of Self-Determination, and under that aegis they ultimately supported the Higashi families' proposal to keep their kids together under one roof. Once they were given the go-ahead, the service provider found a house.

Aside from successfully wrestling the tentacled arms of the group home octopus, I wanted to understand what Robin viewed as the reason the homes succeeded.

"Truly, the stars aligned for us," said Robin, uncharacteristically romantic. "We had the help of the school administration in picking the group of young men to live together, even in helping them choose which bedroom was best: 'Oh, this guy should not be near the laundry room. That guy should be far away from the front door.'" Thus, the school itself was perhaps the keystone to their venture. Higashi has a very strong parent group that gives the parents support as well as offering a speaker series. The school administration has a very positive relationship with the families. And because the house and day program were to be run by the same service provider, the school could help train the staff in both. This makes for a high level of consistency for the residents; staff can overlap and fill in for each other between day program and house, if need be. "It's the house all the staff want to work in," said Robin proudly, "because they are out almost every evening, rock climbing, canoeing."

Advocacy at the state level also played an important role in creating and sustaining the house; Robin's house "had a champion in the DDS, who really helped things work on a systematic level." So even though it feels to Robin that luck and chemistry played a role, the house's success was more about luck guided by good planning. "This is for the long term," said Robin. Over a year later, at the time of writing this book, the house is still highly successful. I recently got together with Robin and she pulled out her phone and showed me a photo of a beautiful engraved award: at their recent annual gala, the service provider gave her son and his roommates a prestigious award of achievement.

Our conversation about Robin's son's group home gave me the opportunity to think back and understand a bit more about why our first attempt at a group house had failed. Even though we took the time to thoughtfully develop a group, our connection was far more nebulous, if not downright superficial or forced. Thinking back, we were mostly just acquaintances from the autism community, and our children had different educational training. And though we tried to get together socially and for the business of discussing group home goals, there was probably not enough of a connection with each other. Possibly we could have chosen a service provider that was more adept at helping families get along, as well as adopting the training methods that were so important to some of the other parents. Higashi had an advantage there because they were all committed to Daily Living Therapy and so could insist on that kind of staff training. Not only did Nat's school not have a deeply connected parent group, they did nothing to help us get to know each other. I had no knowledge of any families of young men who were looking to start a house in the Boston area, and so I did not have that net to fall back on. I had attempted to create my own group from the wider autism family community I had been a part of over Nat's lifetime, but our group did not have the history and solid camaraderie and common experiences that Robin's had.

A Place Called Home: a privately funded, inclusive house

Every state is different in terms of how its DDS works, and its Medicaid waiver availability. Some families end up buying a house as a group. Some incorporate into a nonprofit as a way of controlling the home without any one family actually owning it.

Julie, a mom, educator, and college professor from South Dakota, was one of the first parents I talked to about housing. Together Julie and her husband Tom have created a unique living situation for their thirty-two-year-old son Chris and some friends of his. The home is so successful that Julie has presented their story to many audiences. In their presentation, a Place Called Home is described as "an inclusive group of people with and without disabilities who choose to live together . . . an interdependent community of people who share control and responsibilities." The setting utilizes natural and paid supports for the residents who require this.

Chris is diagnosed with mild to moderate intellectual disability and autism. "Chris needs support," Julie said, "getting showered and dressed, getting breakfast. He's lower functioning in self-care but he has a better social life than I do. He can walk to church and to Augustana [the college nearby]."

When Chris was finishing high school, Julie and Tom felt that he should live as interdependently as possible. At first they thought they would have him live in a group home run by his day program. "It was a beautiful home," Julie said, "built during a window of opportunity when there was federal recovery money from President Obama, during the country's large banking crunch." But that home was to have seven young men with autism, and Julie did not see this as the right setting for Chris. She asked me, "Why would you want seven young men with autism all living together? That's the most unnatural setting that could be." I didn't know what to say, because at the time that was exactly the setting Nat was in. I may not agree with her in that respect: I think that often a group home can run more efficiently if the staff training is geared toward autism and to the particular challenges and similar needs of the group. To Julie, though, it would be more advantageous for Chris to live with people who had complementary needs, so that where one was limited perhaps the other roommates would be more skilled.

Julie and Tom decided that they would set up their own home, but not with the state programs the way I did. They bought the house through an LLC they had formed with Julie's brother. "We have been operating as a family community house. The families share the responsibilities in terms of yard work, cleaning supplies, and other necessary tasks and expenses." This communal sharing of cost and chores was not a difficult challenge for the group. However, having the right attitude—of rolling with what comes up—goes a long way when you go into business with friends and family. Especially very worried autism families. This was something I was learning the hard way; Julie, on the other hand, was wiser than me.

Julie told me that Chris's living situation costs much less than what they'd have to be paying if he were in a state-funded group home. Julie and Tom researched how to maximize federal programs that she could piece together for Chris's home. He qualified for Medicaid, which in his state pays for his rent. Additionally, Chris and his other two roommates have SNAP (Supplemental Nutrition Assistance Program, or food stamps). They also have federal funding for heating assistance in the house during the winter months, which is based on the income levels of the individuals with disabilities that live in the house. The house has thus saved the state a great deal of money when compared to costs associated with existing twenty-four-hour, 365-day group home models. Portions of Chris's Medicaid funding have also been customized to accommodate various individual support services.

The housemates and their families work alongside each other on the physical appearance of the house, specifically to create a good feeling with the neighbors. "A couple of the neighbors already knew Chris and us," explained Julie. "So we baked cookies, talked to them. We had a couple of months to work on the house before we moved in. We baked a pie, chitchatted, and while we did the yard work they'd come over and say, 'Who's moving in?' It worked out really well." Chris did have one neighbor who was very concerned about the snow shoveling, so Julie and the families involved redoubled their efforts to set her at ease. She asked the neighbor, "Who do you use?" And then she hired all of her people. This turned out to be the best way to deal with her. They really had to work at building neighbor relationships and the efforts were worth it, because they earned the goodwill of their immediate community.

Finding people to act as support staff and roommates has been less challenging for her because they live so close to a college campus. Julie and Tom pay graduate students from Augustana College—where Julie teaches—to live at Chris's house and to act as support staff to the three roommates with disabilities. Julie explained that "the three roommates earn money for sleeping at the house, and also for any additional support times they assist Chris, like meals and bedtime routine." Their funding is through the state Medicaid waiver. Most states have Medicaid waiver money for their most involved people with disabilities, but be aware that waiver funds are often limited and you have to advocate hard for them. The waiver guidelines allow Chris and his roommates to choose what they need from their companions. Julie explained, "They live at the house, as we wanted a natural living experience. Each person, including Chris, signs a one-year lease. Some roommates have stayed two years. As far as special training, we have house meetings as needed and when they first move in, we do our own specific 'Chris' training."

Chris also gets support from 3:00–5:00 p.m. after his day program. On weekends, sometimes Julie pays for the support staff's hours—it depends on how much money they have in their budget that month (because Julie manages everything, including all of Chris's allotment).

To Julie, having this kind of control over each aspect of Chris's life is pivotal to his growth. "We're huge proponents of Person-Centered Planning—even before it was a concept," Julie said. Person-Centered Planning is like Self-Determination. Both are favored by most disability advocates these days; its goal is to keep the disabled person's needs and preferences at the forefront of any decision made on his behalf. The disabled person is the author of his own life.

The other piece to Chris's success that Julie has identified is to always think about inclusion. "When he was little, we had a third grader on his IEP team; we wanted that lens. The early days were all about getting him included, not isolated and excluded." Using the nearby college to give Chris access to typical peers—even paying them to be his support staff—is an ingenious way to assure that Chris is a part of his community.

Julie also reminded me that remaining inside the embrace of a community is critical to the health of the family as well. "Networking is so important," Julie concluded. "You have to build a community, people around you and your son or daughter. It is so overwhelming for so many parents. You can do it and succeed if you reach out." Even if you don't end up actually finding your child roommates from your community families, you still need your community—for information and contacts, but, most of all, so that you don't feel alone.

Basically, if you are thinking about creating independent housing for your loved one with autism, you need to sit down with pen and paper and think about what you can do, what works for you. What are your assets? If you are renting a place, and you have very little extra income, you probably need to consider connecting with other, similar families, and perhaps pooling your resources. Or if your loved one wants their own apartment, they will need a resource for their rent. If a separate space is what your autistic loved one needs, don't give up on that.

Private, self-supported farmstead

I'm continually struck by the can-do attitude of some autistic individuals as well as autism parents. What does it take to be able to say to yourself, "Hey, I can do that!" and then go ahead and actually do it? Diane from Pennsylvania was a delight to talk to about her creation, Juniper Hill Farms, because she could laugh about every aspect of her experience there. What made this project work out so well for her?

Probably one of the key factors in Diane's life that prepared her for the challenges of owning a farmstead for autistic adults was the job she had at eighteen as a recreation therapist in the Willowbrook Institution (the infamous institution that journalist Geraldo Rivera ultimately exposed, leading to investigations and the movement to close institutions). Most of that job entailed taking people for walks, swimming trips, parties, dancing, and finding ways to connect with them, yet her exposure to the amazing people with disabilities in her care—their joy and passion for life, even if living in an institution—ultimately sparked her fire to create something different. Diane stayed at Willowbrook for five years.

When Diane moved out West, she worked in a children's group home and there met Brent, a thirteen-year-old with autism. At three years old, his family had given him up to foster care, and he was moved to the group home when he hit puberty. Something clicked between Diane and Brent, and he has been part of Diane's family ever since.

Eventually Diane moved back East and came up with the idea of having a farm; a place that would feel like home to both of them. "I started this farm because both of us loved working on farms so much." With the equity in their family home, she and her husband bought two nearby homes with acreage that had been recently abandoned and combined them to create Juniper Hill Farms. "The two houses are very simple, built in the fifties and sixties. You don't have to have fancy places to live. But they were such a mess when we bought them. The first one Brent [whom she and her husband have adopted] moved into eight to ten years ago took forever to clean up. This year is the first year I've felt like I'm not embarrassed when people come see the farm."

Diane's original idea was to provide housing and be a licensed day program as well. But she quickly realized that it would work better if the farm were a "place to live, and a community of friends." Most of the time the roommates don't want to work where they live; they want to volunteer at an animal rescue, and see other animals—even though there are many animals on Juniper Hill Farms, including angora rabbits, cashmere goats, alpacas, chickens, geese, potbellied pigs, and a "wonderful old donkey." The guys don't want to be on the farm all day because they are isolated enough. All residents are out in the community every day. However, it is required that all residents do farm work.

The residents rent from Diane, and she sees herself as just the landlord—but of course she is so much more. She is the brains and heart behind Juniper Hill Farms. She lives in one of the two houses. "It is not institutional in the least, with five guys in two houses," said Diane. "They have waiver funding personally, but I have nothing to do with it. There are five different waivers here; they're in different systems. The older guys are in the intellectual disability adult system (in their state's equivalent of DDS) while another group of guys is on the physical disability waiver. Their funding pays for staff, transportation, therapy (behaviorist), and coaches."

Diane's goal has been to maintain a "real life" atmosphere. Because the residents rent from Diane, there is a feeling of independence and adult responsibility—no agency taking care of everything for them. This method has worked for several years and with several groups of roommates. Diane cautions, "The only thing to watch for is your township's rules about how many unrelated people can live together. You are almost always OK with three people. I helped set up one house with a landlord who wanted to rent to individuals with disabilities. In that house, everyone has individual leases and the landlord does not hold them accountable if someone leaves . . . it has happened twice, but I helped him to find other housemates."

Diane's projects—such as growing sunflowers and selling crafts made by the residents at a local farmer's market—have so far made enough money for her to expand, and to keep going. The houses she and her husband bought were not expensive, even though they came with a lot of land, because of the bad condition they were in. Diane explained her process, which sounded so common sense, so doable. But it wasn't easy: "They were fixer-uppers. My retired uncle comes each year during warm weather and we pay him to 'fix up' everything . . . he goes back to Arizona when the weather starts to get cold. We purchased our family home twenty-four years ago for $150,000, and then fifteen years later, with the equity we bought the abandoned little two-acre ranch next door for only $65,000, with no mortgage. Five years or so after that, the second house on the lane—where I now live—became abandoned and we got it, with four acres, for $180,000 with a line of credit from our bank because of the equity in the two houses we already had! Rent money from the five guys more than covers the monthly mortgage."

Diane's strategy is so wise and earthy. I believe her success is due in large part to her wonderful attitude, her strong work ethic, and her canny business sense. She is constantly on the lookout for free sources of labor and overlooked properties, and she keeps her expectations reasonable. Like my friend Robin, she credits luck somewhat, but I find that there is so much work and focus, so much adherence to her goals, that luck may have little to do with it. Keeping your sense of priorities is a must, according to Diane: "Everyone needs to accept the idea that the house is going to be simple, without fancy furniture and in-ground swimming pools—this is a huge problem here, in affluent Chester County, PA! Families want their kids to live like they do, instead of like other young people starting out."

I realized the same thing when I was looking for places for Nat to live. I didn't know at first that I was looking for my kind of condo or house, one that was charming and far too expensive. Young adults don't need that kind of thing. Think about where college graduates live when you're looking around for housing.

The makeup of the home

Diane's group home is a mix of guys on the autism spectrum. "Brent is the only one who doesn't talk. Another of the guys has more classic autism, speaks in a lot of scripts. He has Tourette's and obsessive-compulsive disorder. The other guys are more Aspergers." Their challenges have not been obstacles to having good relationships with each other: "If you focus on their day-to-day life, if they develop relationships, they are happy." The young men have to figure out how to get along, how to budget, how to eat healthy enough, how to develop friendships. It's miraculous to Diane how these guys grow. They form deep bonds and feel safe with each other.

When the trust develops, they get through most troubles, and they can even joke about it. Diane said, "They can move on. One of the guys couldn't control tics and outbursts, but now he doesn't have that fear of disapproval, which would escalate him even more. Tourette's is noisy, OCD means that housemate is always moving stuff around. They can now say, 'Oh so-and-so moved it. He's having a hard time,' rather than screaming at him."

This year is the first time Diane feels that things are truly gelling for the group.

The residents don't have a forty-hour work week. "Their anxiety level is too high," explained Diane. They don't need to work fulltime, anyway. "They get the seven hundred dollars a month from SSI, and make a little extra money. Brent crochets. Someone in his group home taught him to crochet years ago, and it is now his preferred method of self-calming. Now they've got him trying to match colors," Diane said. "He has learned that six skeins of yarn is the right size blanket for people to buy. He sells them at the farmer's market for thirty-five dollars."

Another of the young men goes to the library and volunteers at the Lego club. But by far the most unusual job they created at the farm was a pet tombstone business. "One of the older guys who loves dogs also loves cement—they are autistic, after all, and this disability is known for its unusual passions and intense ability to focus," said Diane. "This housemate was making stepping-stones and a person with a dog who had just died saw them and asked, 'Oh, can you make one and put Oreo's name on it?' And a pet gravestone business was born."

For the first three years, once a week on Thursday afternoons the guys had gone as a group to a low-key farmer's market. This year they have cut down on trips to the market to every other week, which is more manageable for them. "We go to the market and have a presence in the community," said Diane. "On a good week we have seventy sunflowers we sell in bouquets with zinnias, and we sit for hours. I pay the guys ten dollars to sit there." This is how the residents make some spending money for themselves.

Thus Diane is able to offer her residents vocational work, pursuits they really love and are good at. Diane was careful to stress that things are by no means perfect for them in terms of how well the farm itself works. "We screwed up this year; the sunflowers got some kind of virus," she said, with her characteristic unflappable attitude.

Diane offered some great advice for getting something off the ground in terms of creating a place like Juniper Hill, and how to help guys like Nat find meaning in their days: "You have to pick what you love if you're with these guys, and I love it. Even in more successful growing years, the time spent in the market is long and tedious—not the glamorous country scene we might all imagine."

Diane is an optimist about the future, even though she can see change is coming. Now Diane is nervous because one of the guys is moving out on his own in a year. They have been so stable that imagining the addition of a new person to the mix is hard. "Everyone wants some kind of stability and to depend on it to last," Diane said. "But there's no such thing. That's why I'm so into relationships. You nurture the relationship and other people have each other's back. When parents pass away, if the person has a community, people rally and the person ends up still living the life that he wanted if the family has set it up well enough."

Diane's words about the importance of relationships apply to all of us. It is the people around us, the community, who ultimately are our saving grace. But we have to cultivate and nurture those bonds within and beyond the immediate group living together. "Throw a party. Get to know your neighbors," Diane suggests. "It takes a few years. Relationships are the key and you just have to build that."

Opting for twenty-two at twenty

I don't always learn what to do next; sometimes I learn what I could have done differently. In that frame of mind, I recently spoke to Cheryl, a friend of mine and the mom of Nicky, an affectionate young man who is social though nonverbal. He frequently seeks out engagement from others in his life. "He's playful," Cheryl told me, her blue-green eyes twinkling. "Nicky is so attuned to others that he goes up to them, looks them right in the eye, nose-to-nose, and says, 'Boo hoo? Boo hoo?' if he senses they are not happy. He can tell how I'm feeling even if I have my back to him," Cheryl said.

During Nicky's teen years, Cheryl worked for a service provider—an organization with offerings such as day programs, after-school activities for children with developmental disabilities, support groups for the families, legal and funding information, and housing options approved by the state's Department of Developmental Services—that was about to open a new group home for some of its clients. The team discussing the home called Cheryl in to a meeting to give them her perspective as a parent. They asked her to talk honestly about Nicky and his needs. Cheryl told them that Nicky is severely impacted by his autism, and that he would need lifelong support. "I'm very afraid of the future," she told the group, "My son will only be able to be in a group home situation because of the level of support he needs." Cheryl knew that Nicky could not live at home because of his high level of aggression. Only a group home would have enough staff to keep him in check.

To Cheryl's surprise, George, the group's liaison looked at her and said, "Excuse me, but how dare you suggest that your son is not capable of being a success anywhere but in a group home?"

Cheryl was taken aback by his tone, but something about his certainty made her control her emotions and think. What was he seeing? How could there be more for Nicky? She could not imagine the answer, and in fact did not have the time or the energy to delve into this new territory just then; however, she knew that she would return to this strange moment later on. She managed to say, "I want to have a conversation with you in the future about what you are talking about . . ."

For the previous few years, in his late teens, Nicky had been in a very restrictive institutionalized hospital residential setting, set up by the public school who determined that his explosive behavior made group homes no longer a possibility.

By the time Nicky was almost twenty, Cheryl had come to believe that Nicky's aggressive outbursts were the result of his frustration with not being understood—particularly at his institutional residential program as well as during school. Cheryl had had enough of the school, but there were no other options for him at that time. He was clearly not progressing there—in fact, the opposite was true. He was communicating through aggression. He required a staffing ratio of 2:1. So Cheryl and her husband, Alex, knew he could not live in their home; they had tried this, and they had seen that they could not handle his intense needs adequately, not without occasionally needing medical attention themselves from Nicky's outbursts. And so when their town's Special Education Director asked them what school they would want if they could transfer, Cheryl told him, "There's no way we're going to find a school at this point . . . it will take a year for them to get to know him." Starting a new school at twenty with only two years to go seemed futile. The IEP team became very concerned that for Nicky turning twenty-two was going to be a brutally challenging transition. Was there any educational and residential solution that would be right for Nicky?

Cheryl flashed back to that irritating but compelling question that George, the agency liaison, had asked her two years before: *How dare you suggest that your son is not capable of being a success anywhere but in a group home?* And now she let herself wonder: what had he meant? What was he thinking of for Nicky? Something opened up for her, a space in her mind where she saw a new possibility: no more hospital programs, no more debilitating group homes. No more school.

She called George, at last. She told him it was time for him to explain what he had meant. George described shared living, in which a disabled person moves into a caregiver's home. For the most part, shared living setups cost less than a bed in a group home for the state DDS. A group home has more levels of compliance standards and oversight, while shared living is less of a bureaucracy and potentially a better quality arrangement. Of course, much depends on finding the right caregiver, but I have found so many families having success with this that I don't believe it to be as difficult as it may seem at first. And remember, with a group home, there is a similar chance of a staff member not working out. In Nat's group homes—the school residence and later the we put one together for him at age twenty-two—we had difficulties maintaining consistent house managers, and new staff cycled in and out. The reality of life is change, even though that can be harder for our autistic guys than it is for more typically developed people. The key is to have adequate transition time, an idea of what sort of living arrangement is needed, and plans to get your child accustomed to it.

At first Cheryl didn't think her son could do this shared living thing. He needed 2:1 in his school program. "He had such dangerous behaviors," she told me. But she also knew that he was feeling terrible in his current situation. The school staff for the most part did not understand him and sought to contain rather than educate him. They would even talk in front of him as if he could not understand. "Never underestimate what Nicky can understand," Cheryl told me. Many autism parents feel that way. Our guys are often still or silent waters, but there is no doubt in our minds that they run deep. But George said, "Well, if you're willing to give it a try we're willing to create a situation that would meet all his needs, keep him safe, and create a wonderful quality of life."

Cheryl felt excited but skeptical. But when she talked to some people who had known Nicky most of his life, she was surprised to find the responses were all the same: they were in favor of shared living for Nicky, rather than starting in a new residential school. And although he needed staff monitoring his behavior at all times, he also valued personal relationships, quiet time, his own space, and being the decision-maker.

Once Cheryl knew she wanted to try shared living for Nicky, she set about making it happen. Even though he was not yet twenty-two. Why not? He wasn't getting anything out of school anyway; she would never allow him to spend two more years there. And at twenty, there was no new school to transfer him to that was worth all the transition hassle, only to graduate at twenty-two and face these questions of placement all over again.

Excited and energized by this burst of new thinking, Cheryl considered her situation. She had years of experience networking. She knew virtually everyone in the disability community and had developed nurturing relationships everywhere. She also lucked out in that their school system's special-education director was a former DDS commissioner, so he knew the state system and had experience with people working out all sorts of situations within its many complex guidelines. He was the only director she knew who was creative and open to unusual solutions. Cheryl and her family found themselves in the perfect storm of expertise, timing, and open-mindedness.

They met with George and developed a team that consisted of the public school system, which funds the student's school placement until the child graduates; the DDS, the state agency overseeing services upon graduation; and various service-providers who offered day programs, day habilitation, and residential options.

They hit a snag when at one point Cheryl wondered how, if Nicky no longer was at the hospital program, would she get him to the doctor, to the dentist—which the hospital staff had always done for her. That was when the DDS case manager referred Nicky to the medical home program through UMass. The medical home program is a multidisciplinary team working together (primary care provider, neuropsychologist, behaviorist, neurologist, psychologist) to take care of all of the client's needs. Very few slots are open for the medical home program, but Nicky's highly competent team got him in.

Cheryl described the medical home model as the following: "In Nicky's case, the first visit was at the doctor's office and it was a disaster; he was very aggressive and destructive. Because of Nicky's clear discomfort with doctors' visits, the team of specialists decided they would have to develop a behavior plan to make him able to tolerate this experience."

First the team start paying brief visits to Nicky at his day program and also at his home. Next, the staff also provided positive behavior reinforcements—a typical method used in helping people with autism learn new skills and more appropriate behaviors. Usually such reinforcements can be things like rewarding the student with favorite foods or preferred activities like a few minutes of shooting baskets, time on the computer, or watching a video.

Nicky learned to tolerate the experience of a doctor's visit, at which point the team slowly begin familiarizing him with short examinations and all the routines involved there—using the stethoscope, thermometer, palpating his abdomen.

The team developed visuals as an additional support—pictures and representational drawings for the routines, which is another popular educational technique for people with autism. Nicky eventually grew comfortable with all of the procedures, and at that point they began bringing him to the doctor's office. Eventually, he was able to attend scheduled appointments with his caregiver and other home staff—but we're getting ahead of ourselves.

The pilot is over, but it proved highly successful. "The team now keeps him as a patient on their regular lists. They coordinate the visits so that each patient who needs to will come to the office to see all the specialists at once, rather than making multiple visits," Cheryl told me. Her new team had proven to be dynamic and solution-oriented.

The transition to shared living took about a year. Because the prior placement situation had been so horrific, they decided that the school would have nothing to do with planning the transition. After all, the school had made him out to be a monster incapable of succeeding in any environment except a hospital, and Cheryl had had enough of that attitude toward Nicky. Especially now that they had the promise of a new, far more supportive living arrangement for him.

Cheryl and Alex decided that they would need to buy a house after considering all of the potential for Nicky damaging things. Buying an entire house? I felt dismayed at hearing this. Who can afford to do that these days? But Cheryl told me it was possible, even for a solid middle class family like hers. In the end, all they had to come up with was a down payment, because their service providing agency would lease the house from them at a price that covered the mortgage. The agency found Isaac (name changed at Cheryl's request), who had been a caregiver for another highly impacted young man for five years and had thus proven his ability to work with someone like Nicky. The arrangement the provider worked out with Cheryl was that Isaac would pay rent to Cheryl's service-providing agency out of his stipend (the stipend is a stipulation of a shared living arrangement), then the agency would give the agreed-upon rent money to Cheryl, while 60 percent of Nicky's Supplemental Security Income (SSI) benefit would cover part of the rent (which is the customary arrangement with Social Security).

Cheryl was able to draw from savings—money not needed for Nicky's college education—for their down payment.

Cheryl and her agency knew that Nicky's transition would require intensive planning because of Nicky's deep-seated need to control whatever he can in his life. Even though he is nonverbal, like any other person he still cares about being able to understand the order of his days. Cheryl told me how he once put his head through a wall in reaction to unanticipated change in his life. While Cheryl talked about this, I recognized in her my own familiar old despair, hammered into steely resolve.

They transitioned him into his new house when Nicky was almost twenty-one. She gave Nicky no advance warning about the move-out. This was a calculated decision because Nicky has a lot of trouble understanding events in the future. Too much anticipation makes him confused and anxious. Nat is very similar in this way.

When the day came, Cheryl and Alex came in with a box to pack Nicky up. Right in front of him, they took things down from his walls, and had Nicky help. When the room was packed up, Cheryl said, "We're all done here." Nicky definitely understood what "all done" meant and he had a grin on his face. He probably had hated the place more than Cheryl had. He helped carry his box out.

To what degree did he really know what was happening? There is no way to know for sure—a sad reality for many autism parents whose children have difficulty communicating—but Cheryl felt that on some level, Nicky was indeed glad to go.

As expected, however, it was a very difficult transition for Nicky at first. But having planned so thoroughly, nothing was a surprise for his parents. They were fully prepared. The shared living provider had budgeted additional funding for a thirty-hour-a-week support person to be in the home with Nicky and the caregiver. Nicky's service providing agency had five additional people on standby for emergency call-ins. This way Cheryl would not be the first person called when there was a problem with Nicky. Even though the beginning of the placement was rocky, within the first year Nicky's aggressive behaviors had dropped by 80 percent. Clearly Nicky had been suffering at his former placement. Cheryl believes that he needed not only to get away from the school but also to have much more freedom.

And ultimately, Nicky also needed a more normal life—one in which he went out into the community, to restaurants, the movies, sporting events, and in which his caregivers understood and liked him. This is what he has found with Isaac.

In terms of communication, Cheryl, Alex, and Nicky's team have found that using www.box.com, where they share notes online, is a good way to keep everyone in the loop, and also to keep their boundaries to keep it all professional. With such tools, there is no going behind anyone's back, a very important factor when dealing with multiple organizations (day program or day hab and the residential service provider).

Relationships between parents and programs can be tricky, and it's best to go in with your eyes open to potential pitfalls. Being too controlling, or going behind people's backs and not being direct—this is the sort of behavior that can destroy relationships. Cheryl warned, "Be careful, because more shared living situations have been destroyed by meddling parents." So far she and her husband have stayed out of it and let the service providing organization do the managing. "I didn't want to become that mom that had to keep coming back and rescuing," she said wisely. (Other families may like more oversight, the degree of which is your choice.)

This did make me wonder about how much more letting go I would have to do over the coming years, because I am definitely a rescuing mom. But one thing at a time.

Lessons Learned About Beginning Post-Twenty-Two Planning

- Start planning early in your child's life. Don't let anyone tell you it's not time yet.
- Jot down ideas and put them in a folder. That's all you need to do for now. Come back to it later. In other words, pace yourself.

- Don't be afraid to ask questions. Ask other parents, ask your Individualized Education Plan team, ask your state's Department of Developmental Services.
- Go to transition-planning workshops, but not too many at a time. Start with your local Arc. (The Arc is a national association of regional support, advocacy experts, and service providers. There are Arc branches all over the country.) See www.thearc.org.
- Try to meet just one person at each workshop and connect with them on Facebook or via email. This is how you start your community of parents. When you find someone who knows about adulthood, stick with them. Meet with them as much as they will put up with you until you understand what you need to do.
- Give yourself time to process what you've learned, and all the emotions attached.

Resources for Housing

- Check out Cheryl's presentation, "Twenty-Two at Twenty: A Nontraditional Transition Story," at www.slideshare.net/cherylryanchan.
- Contact Advocates, Inc. to find out more about their Chinese culture-based group home at www.advocates.org.
- There are websites in each state that guide you within the adult disability services systems. Each state is different, but here is an example of such a website called Disability Benefits 101 in California: www.ca.db101.org/ca/situations/youthanddisability/
- AIDD (Administration on Intellectual and Developmental Disabilities) is a federal government agency that also lists disability resources, state-by-state: www.acl.gov/Programs/AIDD/Prog_Proj_Contacts/index.aspx

- Apply for a Section 8 voucher at the Housing Authority. Section 8 is a federally funded housing program that provides rental assistance to eligible (limited income) people—many people with disabilities have very restricted incomes if they are living on SSI. Section 8 assistance provides eligible participants with alternative housing choices and opportunities to achieve some kind of economic independence and self-sufficiency, according to the federal Mobile Housing website:portal.hud.gov/hudportal/HUD?src=/topics/housing_choice_voucher_program_section_8
- Be sure you have SSI and Medicaid if you qualify: www.ssa.gov/ssi/
- Learn about the ABLE Act and how its passage might benefit your loved one (www.congress.gov/congressional-report/113th-congress/house-report/614/1), and check out this Autism Speaks interpretation: www.autismspeaks.org/news/news-item/10-things-know-about-able-act

Maximizing public programs to create housing

I interviewed Cathy Boyle, a friend, autism mom, and housing expert who was recently appointed by the governor to the Massachusetts Autism Commission, and who founded Autism Housing Pathways, a 501(c)(3) dedicated to helping autism families find housing solutions. Cathy is an expert in that she has looked into so many federal and state programs, and she has also created housing for her son—a publicly funded group home somewhat similar to Robin's, although without an overarching philosophy like the Higashi situation.

Cathy built her process for roommate selection around considerations like staffing ratio needed. She said, "There are three different populations: the Priority One (highest need), who need a

1:1 staffing ratio or thereabouts; the Priority Two (more independent), who need a 1:4 ratio but will not qualify for residential services; and the clients who can do with a 1:8 ratio." It's important for autistic adults and their caregivers to determine what number of staff is necessary for them.

Cathy also pointed out that families must consider what the grouping should be: a mixed group of different genders, different ages, different disabilities? There are no concrete answers to this question; each family must decide for itself what their vision is. In our case, I wanted Nat to be with all young autistic males.

Cathy laid out a few rules of thumb for me, in terms of what every family should do for their autistic family member, before they are even close to twenty-two. I have fleshed out her general advice below, which is laid out in four parts:

1. Save money.
2. Sign up for the relevant support programs.
3. Assemble your guy's peer group or potential roommates.
4. Meet with the Department of Developmental Services with the potential roommates and push for state Medicaid waiver funding.

1. Start saving money when the child is ten years old, or earlier!

Now that the ABLE Act or Achieving a Better Life Experience Act of 2014 has become law, it is possible to save up to $100,000 tax free for your special needs child. According to https://www.congress.gov/bill/113th-congress/house-bill/647, the ABLE ACT is meant "to encourage and assist individuals and families in saving private funds for the purpose of supporting individuals with disabilities to maintain health, independence, and quality of life; and provide secure funding for disability-related expenses of beneficiaries with disabilities that will supplement, but not supplant these individuals' insurance benefits."

2. Sign up for the relevant federal programs.

SSI, Medicaid, and Section 8, which is a federally funded housing program that provides rental assistance to eligible (limited income) people. Section 8 assistance provides eligible participants with alternative housing choices and opportunities to achieve some kind of economic independence and self-sufficiency, according to the federal Mobile Housing website.

The age of eighteen is a milestone for our guys. Cathy talked about Supplemental Security Income, SSI, and Medicaid being the pillars of autism adult services. By eighteen, parents must be sure their autistic loved ones are signed up for SSI and Medicaid. SSI is a benefit through the federal Social Security Administration, paid to disabled adults and children who have limited resources and income. Medicaid is the federal insurance program under the Social Security Administration that allows states to set up home and community based services for the developmentally/intellectually disabled populations (the autism community is often one such recipient).

Exhaust the public funding possibilities.
Cathy emphasized the need to sign up for the federal Section 8 program. "Get him on as many Section 8 voucher waiting lists as possible, ideally at eighteen." There are two kinds of vouchers for housing under Section 8: the *Mobile Voucher,* and the *Project-Based Voucher.* The Mobile Voucher recipient can move anywhere to any Section 8. There is a long waiting list for Mobile Vouchers, and so applicants must be sure to be on the list as soon as they turn eighteen.

The *Project-Based Voucher,* on the other hand, is applied to one particular building or unit, and is restricted to that unit, and does not travel with the recipient. The participant must apply to their local housing authorities for these particular reduced rental units. Look into creating a project-based Section 8 in your town. There are sometimes vouchers available at your local housing authority. Set up a meeting with the housing authority in your town or city; as a taxpaying citizen, it is your right to meet with any city employee. See if you can educate your housing authority about this new need for housing for autistic adults; they may not be aware that they should be offering affordable housing that supports the autism population.

Another idea that Cathy talked about frequently was about maximizing the AFC (Adult Foster/Family Care) program. AFC is a Medicaid-based program available in many states, and it is a funding mechanism that allows a person with a disability to live in the home of a caregiver or caregivers, under their care. The caregiver receives a small stipend for their services. The idea behind AFC is to keep the disabled person in his community rather than in an institution or even a group home.

Cathy came up with a plan that allows a family to maximize their AFC stipend by designating an adult family member to become the Adult Family Care provider and receive a stipend of, for example, about $9,000/year (this is an approximate conservative amount in Massachusetts; it may differ from state to state). The family member saves as much as they can of the Adult Family Care stipend in a separate account. In approximately ten years, the family may have saved $90,000. Even if the family has had to use more than half of that money caring for their autistic loved one in their home, they would still end up with a potential source for a down payment on a privately funded group home or for building on an apartment or extension to your own home (Autism Housing Pathways). To that end, families should also look into any possible low-interest or zero-interest disabled homebuyer loans. Always check with a special needs attorney before moving ahead with these ideas.

3. Get your group together.

At the same time, get a group together whose autistic family members have similar needs and challenges. Find them by connecting at conferences, Special Olympics sporting events, or your loved one's school community. Once you have a group committed to your project, go to the Department of Developmental Services as a group with a plan and a service-providing agency picked out.

4. Meet with the DDS.

Even if you don't have or want a group home, go to the DDS with your plan and the name of the service-providing agency you have selected to work with. Cathy noted that "now that DDS will not be determining eligibility until twenty-two, it may be trickier to create 'out of the box' housing at twenty-two, since you won't be assessed for eligibility until the last minute. Families may need to consider accepting a vacancy in an existing group home from DDS to get into the system, while still working toward creating something that better meets their needs."

An Overall Summary of What Works in Creating Housing

- If possible, use your child's school community and admin-istration as a place to start gathering your group. But look for housemates from all kinds of places.
- Start early in the housemate hunt—socializing, visioning, and planning—possibly as early as sixteen.
- Be sure to save money, but you must consult with a special needs attorney to keep the housing savings account sepa-rate (and set up according to the law).
- Determine any commonalities in staffing approaches: what training do they need, and are there any deal breakers?
- Go as a unit to find a service provider who will commit to the families' preferred training approaches.

- Be sure to look into public funding that can help you buy a group home or build onto your existing home, including Section 8 and AFC, as well as your state Department of Developmental Services.
- If you're willing to purchase a home to convert into the group home for your child, look for property that needs work and consider "sweat equity," so that you are not laying out too much money beforehand. Don't overextend yourself.
- Keep in mind that pocket money may be all the housemates need—and sometimes that money can come from the remainder of an SSI check. To this end, tailor jobs to fit their individual preferred activities.
- Give potential housemates a long time to explore living there, as well as a long adjustment period.
- Try to remain flexible; expect change. As in Juniper Hill Farms' example, the living arrangement might end up so successful that some roommates will move out to live even more on their own. And isn't that the goal, ultimately, for anyone raising a family?

Resources for Creating Housing Solutions

- Autism Housing Pathways is a terrific nonprofit that covers many aspects of housing in Massachusetts. Each state is different, but you can find many ideas and rules of thumb from this site and its blog: www.autismhousing-pathways.net
- The federal Medicaid website outlines what states need to do to set up Adult Family/Foster Care homes: www.medicaid.gov/federal-policy-guidance/downloads/faq-12-27-13-fmap-foster-care-chip.pdf

- Take a look at this terrific resource Julie from South Dakota pointed me to, for how to design homes like a Place Called Home: www.allenshea.com/CIRCL/documents/SingleHouseSLS.pdf
- Look into the Juniper Hill Farms story to get inspiration and actual facts and figures on this sort of project: www.juniperhillfarms.org
- Check out First Place and 3L Place as models of mixed-resident, multi-purpose facilities. First Place has a neurodiverse population of residents (discussed more in depth in Chapter Five as inventive solutions to finding staff). Both offer independent living training and are highly connected to their surrounding communities: www.firstplaceaz.org and www.3lplace.org/living.html

CHAPTER FOUR

STAFFING AND TURNING TO OTHERS

"All of us at some point in our lives need care, and all of us at some point in our lives are caretakers. It could be a returning Iraqi vet, an elder who only sees Meals on Wheels every day. Or a young man with autism like Nat. As a Commonwealth we have to take care of each other."

—*Michael Moloney, Chair of Caring Force*

PERHAPS THE MOST CHALLENGING THING of all in autism adulthood is finding caregivers. But if you think about it, this task has always been a part of our lives with regard to our kids. We always need respite, support, and extra help from others. And so we always need to find good people to do that. We're never just on our own, even if it feels that way a lot of the time. We all have to be able to give our loved one over to someone else's care at some point. And so the other difficult challenge in finding people is that we have to learn to trust others.

In autism adulthood, trust probably comes more easily if your loved one has learned some form of communication. But even without speech you can determine if your guy is comfortable with someone or not. There's no secret answer, of course; it is all about your intuition and experience with him. You know his mannerisms, his communication sounds and looks. Nat cannot always answer "yes" accurately, but when he says "no," he means what he says. But this doesn't mean I haven't had my scares and doubts about people. Some of the young autistic men I know have had their own scary incidents—real abuse. It does happen. Our guys are vulnerable. That's the baseline we start with. Being an autism caregiver means you always have to be ready to pounce on a situation that makes you feel uncomfortable.

That being said, it *is* possible to find great people, people you can trust. I do not believe that it is a horrible world out there. Our experiences with Nat have been very positive for the most part. You have to do your homework with the people you hire, with the people you leave him with, and you have to check in. But hopefully you've always done that anyway. You have to remain deeply connected to the people in his life with frequent phone calls, emails, or visits. I'm connected to Nat, though by no means every day. I touch down just enough to be perhaps an unconscious soft part of Nat's mind.

How does one find great people? In terms of using the staff hired by agencies and service providers in day programs, we can at least be reassured that there have been background checks, references, and some kind of training.

But what about the caregiver who lives with the autistic adult? How do you ascertain skill, instinct, and heart? Experience is right there on the resume. But deciding on a live-in caregiver takes focused interviews and a trial period where you can observe your candidate.

First of all, where do you find potential staff? Sometimes the caregiver comes from an ad you've placed. Sometimes it's on Craigslist, or a college or community board. I have found that it doesn't matter where the applicant comes from; what matters is the background check, references, resume, interview, and, perhaps above all, chemistry.

Nat's caregiver

Our best caregiver situation so far came about fairly naturally, from an ad our service provider had placed on Craigslist. John Excellent came to us first as support when Nat was twenty-two. This was when Nat was living with us, having finished school that month, and was waiting for his housing to be ready. I was not entirely comfortable with John at first. Even though he had direct experience with the autism and adult disabled population from his job at a local service provider, I did not appreciate his opinionated manner. It seemed like he didn't realize he was a new person for Nat. Back then I felt that he should act new and hang back a little, learning from *us* about what worked with Nat.

But John is not like that. Twenty-four years old at the time, full of excitement about his life and dreams (and a little full of himself, I must add with all due affection), he had his own ideas about how to interact with Nat from the very beginning. In his interview, he leaned back on the couch like an old friend, talking in a voice slightly louder than the rest of us. He waxed confident with stories from work and scenarios of what he envisioned for Nat, describing just how he would deal with problems when they came up. Somehow this irritated me because it wasn't what I was expecting. But I'm weird that way. I think that first impressions are often false impressions for me. Sometimes I pay attention to the wrong thing. I expected John to be one way and I was taken aback by the fact that he was not.

We took a chance on him anyway because, other than his strong gregariousness, he did have so many great qualifications and ideas. It turned out that John's comfort and confidence were his best qualities. His certainty about his own abilities and about what worked with Nat ended up being his strength, something he could rely on in the tough days to come. John ended up moving with Nat to his first adult house as an aide there, and then to the group home that I had helped set up with friends. He eventually became the house manager at that home.

So I decided to ask John—whom I now consider an expert on Nat and caregiving in general—to tell me his thoughts and philosophies about working as a caregiver, hiring, and training support staff.

"It all comes down to passion," he said, his words carrying just a whisper of a Haitian French accent, "because it's not the best pay in the human services field. What I do when I interview staff is look for people who are passionate, and who want a career. Generally I find two kinds of staff: one who looks at this as a job, and one who sees this as a steppingstone. They want to climb up the ladder—not only do they want to learn, they want to make sure that what they do is fulfilling, and that they are making a difference. I would rather get a staff person who is completely inexperienced but open-minded and passionate than a staff person who is in the same job for ten plus years. I wonder, if they're so experienced, why haven't they taken the next step? With autism it doesn't necessarily matter how many years' experience you have."

John explained his process in choosing prospective candidates to interview: "When I look at a resume, I look at what they are studying if they're in college. Then I'll talk to them and kind of get a vibe off of what they say and how they say it. I look for some key words." When John interviewed Uja, a candidate for Nat's home—and one of the finest workers and people I have ever met—Uja had said, "Well, I have a calm personality." That showed John a certain self-awareness and the right temperament for the job. "With these individuals, if you are a very vibrant over-the-top type you can actually bring up an autistic person's level of anxiety," John said. Actually, John has a healthy degree of vibrancy of his own. He always wears bright Caribbean colors; his laughter is surprising, sudden, and belly-deep. One Halloween he strode in wearing a rainbow derby, suspenders, and bow tie—during the day, for one of Nat's doctor's appointments! Nat was also dressed up, in a Mad Hatter–style hat and sunglasses.

Based on my observations of John, I did not share the viewpoint that actively enthusiastic people can cause Nat anxiety. This is not something I have found to be true. In fact, Ned and I used to always look for what we called "over-caffeinated" staff when we hired people to work with Nat after school. We thought that he needed people with marked enthusiasm to pull him out of himself a bit.

But this kind of disagreement is what happened when I first met John. This is what made me uncomfortable—at first. But what I realized was that John saw things differently from me, and he had the ability to back up his observations. Eventually, I saw that he made a lot of sense. I had to admit that, in fact, I have found that if I *lower* my voice with Nat to almost a whisper, he will then hear me.

John looks for good communicators. "Lack of communication is one of the biggest problems in living situations," John said. "It works well when you have a well-oiled machine where all the staff is communicating and things are being done. Then the residents are happy and doing what they're supposed to do. When there is a setback, then staff knows how to handle the situation; for example, if a resident has an anxiety behavior, staff should know how to calm the person down. The staff should know what the individual is trying to tell them. Then, as the manager, I feel I can be absent from the job without going crazy worrying about the guys." John told me that in general, when working with autistic people, preparation for any change was key. This may come as no surprise to autism families. The surprise, however, is hearing the extent to which John and his staff prepared for the group's move. Nat's group at that point was on its third physical location. The first arrangement had deteriorated because the families could not agree with the family who owned the house. The second arrangement was a temporary one, until a new building was found.

Once the service provider bought the new house, getting it ready took longer than we all expected. This was a source of anxiety for the families, because we worried that it would be very unsettling for our guys. We were also angry with the service provider for taking so long to find a house. This may have been a bit unfair because buying a house in Boston is never easy, and the DDS had so many requirements (a back egress on every floor, low price range) that the delay is completely understandable. John described what he'd done to remedy the tension for the guys.

> *I had a countdown schedule. The guys brought in their personal effects into the new home and hung stuff up as a transitional step. In the end everyone knew they were moving March 7. Then, the night before the move-in, I found out that the house wasn't ready. They couldn't get the inspector there in time to sign off on all the changes. I went in and did a little more transitional stuff with the guys. The next day I was late coming in, and all the individuals were really upset and anxious. Some of them were starting to scream and just walk around and around—a sure sign of coming outbursts. As I came in, however, I saw the two staff kind of separate the guys and each chose the guy they were most effective with. Then a third staff ended up coming in just because he knew the staff needed support without even moving! I ended up stepping in to help, but actually the staff was able to handle everything just fine without me.*

This, to John, is the best kind of success.

Training is thorny. Not just because you can never tell if a staff person has really internalized the approach, but also because these are all human beings we're talking about—staff as well as clients—and you never know if an approach is the "right" one. People change all the time.

John thinks of training in a characteristically down-to-earth way. Knowing about autism is important, of course, but knowing the autistic clients themselves is key. John gives the clients plenty of advance notice for anything or anyone new or different. "I tell the clients 'so-and-so is going to work with you, so you have to be a little more patient.'"

Relationships, whether between a caregiver and a person who has a disability, or anyone else, are a two-way street. Perhaps this is the key to John's great track record with Nat. As much as I hate to say it, too often we neurotypicals sometimes forget that our autistic loved ones are full-blown people, with all the quirks, irritations, emotions, flaws, hopes, and dreams that we have. Accordingly, John fully expects the individuals to do their part to form a successful relationship with the staff, to the extent they can. "Both the individuals and the staff have to be patient," he said. "It's easy for me to hear a client make a particular noise, for example, and know what he wants. He has to get to a point where he may be able to think (on some level): 'you don't know me so I have to be patient. I have to be able to repeat things or to show you things for you to understand.'" John does a lot of work with the residents to explain to them what their role is. "It's not easy," he said. No kidding.

John Excellent's Tips for Transitioning in New Workers

- When interviewing potential staff, be sure to bring the residents into the process at whatever time is most beneficial to them.
- When the staff come for training, let the guys know new workers are coming in to meet them.
- On the first day, be on site to initiate introductions.
- At the end of the training, let the autistic residents know when the training period is over. Hold the individuals and the staff to the same standard. Both parties need to be open-minded. Come in and lend a hand and mediate and help keep the transition smooth.

Determining your own parameters for your staff

Almost from the beginning of my life as Nat's mom, I have turned to other autism parents (and later on, autistic people) for crash courses in what to do next for Nat. Most often I have found my experts on the sidelines of Special Olympics practice, but once in a while I meet a disabilities rock star at a workshop or conference. Mike is in the latter group. Although his son Zack does not have a diagnosis of autism, he does have some similar challenges. Mike has been leading monthly meetings for mostly parents of transition-age kids with autism for around ten years. He is practiced in the science of adulthood for people with intellectual disabilities, and he's also in the financial consulting business. He does not charge for his monthly workshops, and he has sat down with me for coffee and an information session numerous times. Like Jeff Keilson, he is another one of these people whose knowledge is only exceeded by his open heart. By and large, this kind of beneficence is more common than not in my world—though Jeff and Mike are still rarities in the depth of their commitment to others.

Nat was almost twenty-six when I began wondering what other parents did to give their children residential supports if they did not have a state-funded residential arrangement like Nat's. The majority of adults with autism will not have that level of funding in the coming years, due to the higher numbers of people entering the adulthood system. So how involved were other families in finding caregivers for their autistic family members? Did any of the families I know have a system for securing a great provider for their son or daughter?

I got to talking to Mike at a qualifying tournament for our sons' flag football team, and he mentioned that Zack's caregivers only stay with him for a year—and that this "term limit" is Mike's idea, based on experience. "They get jaded after a year," Mike said.

I was fascinated with the idea of deciding ahead of time to put a limit on a caregiver's term. I had always felt at the mercy of rapid turnover, and the fear of good staff quitting or moving on too soon. A lot of parents have anxiety over this, starting in their child's earliest school days, where the turnover rate of special needs staff is mind-boggling and often heartbreaking. Once our guys get used to working with someone, transitioning to another is nearly always a difficult task. It can take Nat up to six months to express his discomfort with a new situation in his life.

But Mike intentionally cuts his staff after one year. How, then, did he find replacements this regularly? We continued our conversation over email. I asked him if he could describe his thinking and his process for finding and working with caregivers.

Typical of Mike, he framed his answer in an organized manner that could help not only me but also others: "All our kids are different, and one solution may be right for one, and not for another. Like all of the other families, my wife and I have never done this before, so we learn as we go. We are heading into our fifth year with Zack 'on his own' and are lucky to have made it this far without any 'major' catastrophes." This kind of success is fairly miraculous, especially for such a newcomer to adulthood.

For Mike, his process comes down to three characteristics: trustworthiness, current life occupation and mindset, and the ability to connect and sustain a healthy and professional friendship with Zack. (Zack lives with another young man, also developmentally disabled, and so this roommate and his parents are also part of the interviewing and decision-making.) I asked Mike about Zack's involvement in the process. It has always been important to Mike that Zack design his own life to the greatest degree possible. He wrote, "Zack is a part of it once my wife and I, and his roommate's family, have agreed on a candidate. We always have them meet the boys so they can all express their sentiments. Usually, the boys are pretty silent about the whole process and are happy to accept whomever we choose. Incidentally, we have learned that Zack likes pretty, young girls for caregivers (who can blame him?)!"

Mike said that he has "no special process other than I always have my antenna up, and the next caregiver is always on my mind." He has discovered excellent potential support for Zach through his family network. "Finding potential staff through existing relationships is almost always the best because you have some sense of their parents and how they were raised," he wrote. He also uses college bulletin boards and applies to www.care.com, a website that finds candidates for a variety of needs, from infant care to elder care to pet care (more about this particular resource later on in the chapter). "Like any vetting process, it generally starts on the phone, and then usually a dinner, and then one last meeting to answer everyone's questions. The boys and/or the parents are present at the dinner, and the boys are always present at the 'final' meeting," Mike explained.

Zack's funding for caregiving support is through the Adult Family Care (AFC) program. The financial allotments are not as comprehensive as state funding through a waiver, but neither are the AFC caregiver's responsibilities. Where Nat's rent and staff salary are covered, an AFC caregiver receives a stipend that helps with expenses. AFC is a great option for people with needs that are less severe than someone like Nat. An AFC client can be someone who needs *some* support in physical self-care, independent living skills, personal healthcare, and in-home safety. In the AFC arrangement, the person with a disability lives in the home with a caregiver or caregivers, under their care.

Although this description may sounds roughly like the support Nat has from our state Department of Developmental Services, AFC is considered much more a part of the community. AFC arrangements are not like a group home; they are a roommate kind of situation. The AFC caregiver is responsible for the individual, but that individual is often out of the house Monday through Friday until mid-afternoon, giving the caregiver a lot of flexibility to pursue classes, additional jobs, and anything else.

The way AFC works is that a service-providing agency conducts interviews and evaluations of the disabled client. They make a determination as to eligibility based on level of help needed, and then the agency, the guardian, or the client himself finds an approved caregiver to live with. Like us, Mike is working with such an agency to administrate the nuts and bolts of Zack's AFC arrangement. But unlike Ned and me—we require more administration and guidance for Nat—Mike chooses to have the service providing agency enter into the process later, once the two families are certain about a candidate. Then the agency steps in and does background checks. Once the caregiver is hired, Mike sets up a kind of adjustment period: "They do an overnight so they can get a sense of the boys' morning routine." Other than that, the families make sure that the new caregiver understands that he or she is only under contract for a year. Mike has found that a year is an excellent length of time for the kind of caregivers he prefers—young adults just starting out from college. Because young adults often decide year by year what they are doing with their lives, this term limit has mostly worked out very well. "The third caregiver wanted to stay on a second year, but we did not allow this," Mike wrote. "She was doing an adequate job, but her relationship with Zack was deteriorating to the point of often being adversarial, which was not acceptable. It was not horrible, but it was not something we would continue." So far they have found that those who have stayed on a second year have not been as enthusiastic in the second year, despite good intentions.

"Creating an end date puts you in a position that there is a reasonable expectation they will stay that long. It puts you in the driver's seat so you are not sitting on pins and needles wondering how long they will stay," Mike wrote. He and I both know all about those pins and needles; most special needs parents live with an underlying anxiety that any good staff person will leave for greener pastures all too soon. Mike's system gives the parent some control over this. A year doesn't feel too long to many people; indeed it may fit perfectly with the lifestyle of the year-by-year graduate student. Thus Mike's one-year stipulation helps them commit and give it their all.

Once a family has determined that the fit is a good one given the three qualifications Mike looks for, he has to make sure that the caregiver is in the right phase of life for the arrangement. The interviews must ascertain whether the candidate can indeed commit to sharing his home and being ultimately responsible for the individuals.

Mike describes his caregiver's duties and the AFC expectations thus:

> *The caregiver lives there full time. It is his/her home. In our case, it is a three bedroom-apartment. Each boy has their own bedroom, and the caregiver resides in the master bedroom with his/her own bathroom.*
>
> *Everyone in the apartment is free to invite their friends and use the apartment as if it were their own, just as the boys can, so long as everyone respects each other's needs/feelings/space. For instance, the current caregiver had a Halloween party at the apartment one Saturday night. She invited her partner and friends. They made pizza and brownies and everyone (including Zack) watched a movie.*
>
> *The caregiver makes sure the boys get off in the morning having been groomed and fed (the boys are able to make their own breakfast). She also makes sure they have made their lunch the night before which they eat at work. She prepares the boys' dinner each night, and in Zack's case makes sure he showers and gets to bed at a reasonable time so he can awake each day (5:30 a.m.). She keeps both guys on schedule and makes sure they do their chores (clean the apartment and do their laundry).*
>
> *The caregiver is free to come and go as she pleases so long as the boys have what they need. Both boys are able to stay by themselves for a period of time. They know how to be safe.*

Bottom line is, Zack and his parents want to be sure that what they have is a real home. This can only happen if the caregiver is trustworthy, qualified, enthusiastic, and able to commit. Mike's system may be the best insurance families can have that each year will be one of growth, safety, and happiness. So far, so good. In the world of autism adulthood, that is a rave review.

Sometimes the best staff is right under your nose

Sue's son Ed found a successful shared living situation with Kathy, a family friend and neighbor for fifteen years. It took them a long time to realize that one great solution for a caregiver for Ed was such a simple and obvious one.

When Sue and Kathy first met, Sue was working at the Autism Resource Center in Massachusetts, and Kathy was a member there. Sue used to take her son Ed to the Center's camp, and Kathy also came with her family. "Ed just gravitated to Kathy. He liked her. I'd be like 'OK, I got Ed's lunch, where is he?' And he'd be with Kathy. He was already sitting at her table and she would be feeding him."

When he turned twenty-two, Ed was approved for shared living, but they could not find a provider (someone to live with him 24/7). For nearly two years, Ed lived at home and Sue drove him to his program every day. But Sue was challenged by picking Ed up on time. "I knew that Kathy drove past the building, and she would stop and pick up Ed and hold him till I got there. I asked her if she'd like to make some money, and she said, 'sure.' We started hanging out at her house," Sue said.

Then the agency that served Ed approached Sue because they had an opening in a group home. Sue didn't want Ed in a group home, but she was afraid to say no and lose his priority with them. "I looked at the home. The other residents were older—in their forties—but he was living with people older than that now anyway—my husband and me. So I said yes."

Ed would visit his parents on the weekends. He was not terribly happy in the group home. Two of the guys were non-verbal, screaming all the time. The other was verbal but sang at the top of his lungs all day. Sue said, "Poor Ed was in his room with his hands over his ears. Ed was higher functioning than the others. Then came the straw that broke the camel's back. One day I picked him up and there was a horrendous smell coming from him, like feces. I took off his sweater and washed it, and also his underwear, which hadn't been changed in days." This was not the only thing amiss, unfortunately. "When I got him back to the group home I decided to go make Ed's bed. I looked at the sheet and there were stains. I went into the closet; I had bought him new sheets, and they were just sitting there in the wrapper. The staff had assumed—because he was capable—that he was stripping his bed himself. But he needed prompts to do that."

Sue is experienced enough with disability workers from her work at the Autism Resource Center that she did not get angry with the staff. She understood the other guys were high-need. She knew the staff were good people, just overwhelmed with the other guys in that house. They were so busy. But Ed was suffering from benign neglect because he was more capable than the others. No malfeasance was involved, just a symptom of a mismatch and an overburdened system of care. Alerting the agency to her findings resulted in more attention for Ed, but she knew that a group home was not the right fit for him.

At last the agency found a home for Ed, a shared living situation, with a couple who appeared well-suited to that lifestyle. "They were great," Sue said. "One of the pair had worked at an agency, and the other had done a lot of respite work. But ten months later, things happened in their lives and they couldn't do it anymore. He was sort of homeless for two months, temporarily living with another shared living provider."

Sue's natural humor ended up saving the day. "At that point I jokingly threw out a remark on Facebook, asking if anyone wanted to take care of a gentle giant, free to a good home." The housing stars were aligned for Ed at last. Kathy answered right away, "We want him. He's like family to us." So he moved in with Kathy and her three sons, who saw Ed as a brother.

Even though this arrangement did recently come to an end—as does everything in this life—for a very long time it was pretty perfect for Ed. And Kathy and her loving family had been right there all along. We all need to keep our eyes open for natural and sometimes obvious potential caregivers.

Finding staff for a farmstead

In Chapter Three, I described Diane's set up at Juniper Hill Farms. Diane has had a lot of success finding staff for her farmhouses. She has a good formula: keeping them a part of the vision, so they stay invested in the house's success. "Some of the staff have been there for four years, the other half for two, so the turnover has been low. This is a key factor in an organization's success—to have everyone invested in the mission, in the group. Everyone brainstorms together. Most of the volunteer positions work out really well. Most people are really receptive."

Diane suggested that her model could work in slightly different ways, where perhaps a family with the means could buy a house with a few bedrooms (like my friend Cheryl from Massachusetts did, also described in Chapter Three) and become the landlords themselves, and then look for tenants that were compatible. The parents in some cases could provide natural overnight support in case of emergency.

But finding non-family staff takes a bit of perseverance and creativity. Diane said, "We actually have advertised on Craigslist and have gotten some amazing applicants; most often they are mature women who have grown families . . . no spouse . . . have sold the family home. In one situation we had six GREAT applicants, all women over forty-five . . . and one applicant that the families hired is still living with the family five years later as an in-home caregiver." You can't ask for a better situation that that.

Jeff Keilson, Cofounder of Rewarding Work

As I've described throughout this book, Jeff Keilson has been a guiding force in my life with Nat as an adult. One of Jeff's causes is helping disabled consumers and their families find staff. To that end, Jeff is cofounder of a nonprofit called Rewarding Work. Jeff told me, "There are more than 22,000 people who require personal care attendants (PCA) in Massachusetts. Some use family, friends, neighbors, their own network. Those who don't have that network need help in finding PCAs. The state is funding Rewarding Work to provide the registry. This is a user-friendly medium to find a worker." Rewarding Work is not yet nationwide. They have a limited reach, but they are still a resource worth considering. For example, they have a database with six to seven thousand workers in Massachusetts. Rewarding Work also has contracts in Vermont, Rhode Island, Connecticut, New Hampshire, and Arizona. Rewarding Work works with people on Medicaid/Medicare.

Rewarding Work does not perform background checks on people before they are listed in the database. They are a nonprofit, so don't have the funds or staff to perform preliminary checks. Jeff said, "You go through with the checks at the point of hire." Rewarding Work provides a link to Massachusetts's Criminal Offender Record Information (CORI) on its site.

Applicants describe their experiences working with disabilities or diseases, what they're interested in doing, whether they want to work with children, adults, or elders, and what hours they prefer. This is the sort of information that helps people sort through the database.

In Massachusetts, anyone on MassHealth can access this service for free. Those who are not eligible for MassHealth can pay ten dollars per month and up to ninety dollars a year to access the site. Currently there's a national effort afoot in terms of gathering a pool of caregivers. Lifespan Coalition of Massachusetts now has some federally funded sister organizations in other states around the country—Arizona and New Hampshire, for example—to focus in on respite workers. In Massachusetts, with the support of the Department of Developmental Services and the Lifespan Respite Coalition, Rewarding Work has expanded to include respite workers. Of course, every state is different in terms of helping consumers find staff.

Jeff's nonprofit has its limitations. "Where the implementation of Rewarding Work falls short is that there are not enough resources dedicated to recruit people who are interested in becoming respite, PCA, and other direct support providers. We have to partner with organizations like community colleges to advertise for applicants." In terms of providing incentives to people who might want to work as PCAs, state agencies and organizations like Rewarding Work have to be creative. "Once a year, the Commonwealth of Massachusetts, in collaboration with Rewarding Work and Service Employees International Union, holds a big event at the State House where awards are given for PCA of the year, chosen from five different regions across the state, as an incentive to workers," Jeff said.

One caveat is that rate-setting practice can be inconsistent. One can possibly get their potential caregiver a stipend from the state and sometimes the client can set the salary, the hourly rate, and pay what they want. Maybe the client sets an even higher than normal pay rate, and chooses to have fewer hours. This ability, this freedom of choice is part of the Self-Determination philosophy, giving the client ultimate control. Of course, sometimes the state or the agency working with the client may be the ones determining the pay rate. But it's always worth asking if it's possible to take control of this aspect. "As we move toward more

Self-Determination, we need a system that is more supportive of that kind of freedom of choice," Jeff said.

Many of the care-finder organizations like Rewarding Work and Care.com provide not only staff resources, but also interviewing tips. Care.com is an excellent resource in general for finding any kind of staff, from special needs support to nannies to dog walkers, for a monthly fee. I tried it out to find someone for Nat (to give John respite) and got several good leads within hours of applying.

It is important to bear in mind that college or masters degrees may not mean much in terms of workers' abilities. One of the best people ever to work with Nat was a Boston University undergrad with no experience whatsoever. She taught Nat to read. Another talented worker was a drama major at Emerson College in Boston. She coached Nat for his first experience in Special Olympics during one of his particularly challenging and aggressive phases. In the end, he never tried to hurt her, she never asked for payment, and he ended up going to the State Games and winning a medal.

Lack of experience can work if the staff person has the right instincts and attitude, but one has to be careful and keep in mind the client's specific challenges. Jeff agreed: "If someone has complex medical needs, [hiring an untrained person] may not be the best idea."

Something additional to be aware of is the issue of stress on caregivers. "There's a huge cost in the employees' health," Jeff explained. "There's also an issue of adequate pay and benefits. The overall low pay sends a signal that the worker is not valued much. That's a huge challenge. How do you get a workforce when the number of available workers for people who need support is going down?"

Ideas on the horizon: Caring Force, Inc.

Michael Moloney is the statewide chair of Caring Force, a movement launched by the Providers, Council (the largest human services trade organization in Massachusetts) that is all about finding solutions for the increasing shortage of caregivers and disability support staff. Caring Force also works toward better pay for these groups, almost none of whom make a living wage: "The people who receive services do better than the people giving services." Mike pointed out how caregivers are often immigrants from other countries, yet they have to get medication certifications, pass CORI and background checks—these are the people who feed, bathe, take care of people in a mental health crisis, yet they work two and three jobs to make ends meet, and they do not get the respect they deserve. "It's just not morally right," Mike said. So he and some of the nearly 20,000 other members of the Caring Force travel around the state meeting with politicians and other leaders, pushing for awareness and action on these workforce issues. Mike told me how the Caring Force was started, illustrating the ongoing need for strong voices at the government level. "We were meeting with the Senate President a few years back, and were talking about staff, and how they don't get the money or respect they deserve. She advised us to get 'on the books,'" meaning, they needed to become a louder presence in the minds of Beacon Hill, those who create the state budget. This turned out to be excellent advice. "We realized then that we needed to have a different way of approaching the legislature. Mobilize thousands of people instead of guys in suits. We actually had so many at one rally that we shut down the State House in 2011."

Mike told me that there's going to be the need for a 60 percent increase in the caregiver workforce by 2022. "It's just going up as the population ages and there are more people with autism and others needing care." To this end, Mike and other visionaries like him have started to come up with an entire menu of possible living arrangements for people with disabilities who will need a lot of care. But the thinking about housing and care options will need to change. The publicly funded group home, for example, is not sustainable in the long run, according to Mike. "Staffing is the culprit. It's one shift after another." Group home costs are exorbitant because of the rotating shifts, required staffing, and overtime. Additionally, a resident of a group home may end up having perhaps 125 caretakers in the course of a lifetime because of the turnover.

Nat used to be in a group home, and I remember how many people were there at any given time. Two staff for five guys, 24/7. And even though the house was in a regular neighborhood, there was very little community interaction. If one guy had a meltdown, sometimes they had to scrap whatever activity they had planned. And certainly they rarely even spoke to neighbors—it was a busy street near a quarry, noisy, with few stores to walk to. People kept to themselves. Sometimes his house felt like a small institution.

Mike said, "I prefer shared living to a group home because it doesn't have shift staffing. Shared living, because of the level of the stipend, is going to become more appealing to people because they will earn $35,000 or more tax free, as well as a place to live. However, the relationship can't be about money; instead, it's about matching people with similar interests." Mike has found that many people will welcome roommates with disabilities if they're asked.

Even though programs like Shared Living likely vary from state to state, it is something for parents and self-advocates to keep in mind. Nationwide, 30 percent of those in need of care are in shared living situations, according to Mike's data.

It is important to ask your state agency if this option is a possibility. Shared living is not an easy arrangement to undertake. There must be a lot of time given to plan and develop all aspects of the living situation. If well-designed, sometimes these arrangements can last a dozen years or longer with the same caregiver. Even when the caregiver moves on, sometime the caregiver's family takes over.

As I mentioned previously, Adult Foster Care (AFC, a program that provides a small stipend to a live-in caregiver) is sometimes an option available through Medicaid. Before I knew if Nat had sufficient residential funding, I had explored staffing an apartment for him through the Adult Foster Care program. If you pursue an AFC arrangement, sometimes your state's Department of Developmental Services can augment the funding with what is called a "wrap-around," i.e. additional money for various supports in conjunction with AFC, such as staff (although usually wraparound funds are not supposed to cover residential staff, but rather to hire people for supports like travel-training staff or community skills-training staff). But to access resources like AFC and wraparound, *you have to know about it to know to ask about it.* The parent, guardian, or self-advocate has to ask first. Don't expect Medicaid—or any other agency office—to come to you offering programs.

At the same time, the programs and those who work for them are not the bad guys. Politics and limited funds are. "Medicaid is under attack now," said Mike, reminding us that we always need to remain vigilant with our legislators, and advocate in order to keep these programs strong.

Mike and other advocates continue to try to improve residential workforce issues in creative ways. One current approach is to get zoning changes so that families could put an addition on their house to provide separate living space for a caregiver. Mike is also exploring the concept of creating cooperative-style complexes with people with autism scattered throughout, living among typical people who have a vocation for caregiving.

Mike pointed out that these creative arrangements could solve two problems at once. One such idea advocacy groups are discussing is to turn to veterans who have recently come back from service. Many often need housing. "Maybe they could be part of a community like this, and do some caregiving in return for housing," said Mike.

Combining higher education and dorm life with independent living skills

Colleges and universities are a gold mine for finding potential staff, a natural workforce. For example, in Massachusetts, Stonehill College offers a program called House of Possibilities, which is actually a day habilitation program. Using this example, you could develop naturally occurring pockets of in-kind mutually beneficial arrangements. You could conceivably create and staff a group home on a college campus, or have shared living apartments scattered in among student housing. Students going into the field could do internships as caregivers, or simply earn extra income. "Right now there are 35,000 college students in Worcester, Massachusetts," Mike said. "How do you leverage that? Not to mention all the other resources at the college, such as the gym, the pool—and it's already an integrated community."

Taft College in Bakersfield, California, was one of the first higher education institutions to dedicate resources to mixed-resident (disabled and non-disabled) housing and curricula. Their Transition to Independent Living (TIL) program is the brainchild of their former Director of Student Support Jeff Ross, a veteran educator, colleague, and friend of mine.

The TIL website's mission states: "The Transition to Independent Living Program endeavors to provide an environment with: enriching collegiate experiences; interactive and inclusive environments; learning outcomes transferable to life-long productivity; career education resulting in gainful employment; self-determination and knowledge of individual strengths; and empowerment through education" (http://www.taftcollege. edu/tcwp/til/).

TIL has thirty-two dorms available, with an incredible dedication to supports: "Staff for the TIL program include administrative, certificated and classified staff. The program maintains a staff ratio of 3:1." With twenty years under its belt, TIL has been able to promise and deliver on independent living and job training for its students. Their data on successful students, even ten years after leaving the program, is very impressive.

Considerations for Choosing Caregivers

- Versatility
- Good instincts
- Ability to read body language

- Ability to help the individuals communicate
- His/her type and degree of experience
- Your comfort level
- The match with the particular needs of your loved one
- Whether this is a raw material employee—someone who needs training. It's easier to train someone to have a particular skill than to train them to have compassion.
- Initials after one's name doesn't translate to a quality staff.

Tips for Organizing Your Search

- If your loved one is not eligible for state waiver funding (which is increasingly becoming the case), Google search words like "personal care attendant" or "adult foster care."
- Set small goals to learn one thing at a time, like this:
- Today I will look for PCA benefits.
- Tomorrow I will look for job supports.
- Then I will call the Social Security Office near me and make an appointment.

Resources for Finding Staff

- Look for people who may have more than a vocation for working with adults with autism; some want to live with our guys and be a complete part of their lives. Check out communities like First Place (www.firstplaceaz.org), Camphill (www.camphill.net), and 3L Place (www.3lplace.org) and ask where their staff comes from. (I believe in "poaching" staff sometimes if you can, by offering them better pay or some other benefit, like room and board or a parking space. Caregiving, like any other work, is a competitive field. All's fair in love, war, and autism.)

- Sometimes college can be a place where designated peers work (and live) with autistic students (like TIL). For a list of organizations devoted to making autism-friendly college experiences, such as College Steps, see: www.collegesteps.org and the College Internship Program (CIP), www.cipworldwide.org.
- Look into services like Care.com and Rewarding Work who specialize in finding caregivers.
- Advertise in places like Craigslist and on college employment boards, as well as at religious institutions for people who may have a vocation for caregiving.

PART II

DECONSTRUCTING AUTISM ADULTHOOD

CHAPTER FIVE

HELPING YOUR GUY FIND HIS WAY

Acquiring Life Skills

"If Carson were not autistic, he would be totally out-of-the-closet gay. We're on the lookout for signs, and how to make him comfortable with it. I really do think he has some insight into what it is to be gay. He loves to get mani-pedis, and picks colors he's seen on Katy Perry and Johnny Depp."

—Donna, mother of Carson, a recently out
gay autistic man

Nothing lasts forever, especially in autism adulthood. It's as if the battles for services during the school years are the way we build up muscle. But autism adulthood requires that we stay in shape, and never allow for arthritic complacency. Old as we inevitably become, we are in no way finished when our guys become adults.

To return to Nat's second group home endeavor: another family joined us, and now we were four. The house was full, but something was missing. Perhaps we had had too many ups and downs and interpersonal troubles that had soured things. We had our same holiday get-togethers, but conversations were a little forced; something was in the air. Still, the staff were committed to us, the guys had a good roof over their heads. Ned and I continued our same routine of taking Nat home on the weekends and trying to fill his time productively with his social group and sports. But I felt like we were going through the motions; the warmth was gone, the sense of community, over.

One day I was sitting in a doctor's office with Nat and Yonel, a staff person in the group home, while waiting for one of Nat's doctors. When you're involved with a state-run group home, staff is responsible for taking the residents to their doctors and there are pages of forms to be filled out each time. But I always come along. By now, three years into Nat's formal adulthood, I was used to sitting with staff and shooting the breeze. I was very comfortable with Yonel in particular, who had been with us since the transition home.

Out of the blue, Yonel said, "You know, I think Nat might do better in an apartment, in shared living."

It was a shock, and yet, it was an idea that burst open in my mind, fully bloomed, like a flower after a lot of rain. Shared living! Nat would be in an apartment. An urban location, like where he'd grown up. Just him and one other roommate: his caregiver. In my mind it seemed like such a fresh idea, a cool breeze in the middle of hot humid August—it would be flexible, and more natural than the group home.

"Really?" I said, letting all my old pictures of it tumble in my brain. The apartment in one of the student neighborhoods, the walks to nearby shops, the rides on the T, Boston's subway system. No need for a van, or for tight staff ratios. A change in living arrangements as momentous as this could lead Nat to a whole new level in experiences and living skills: for example, apartment life with one roommate is a very natural, intimate situation, as opposed to the more impersonal dynamic of rotating staff.

Yonel broke in on my thoughts. "Well, Nat does sometimes miss out on outings because one roommate or another is having trouble, and so they all have to stay home because of that." This was a problem I had wondered about, and it irritated me to hear a staff person admit that this is indeed what happened. So Nat was falling through the cracks because he was in need of less support. It did not seem fair.

An apartment with a caregiver would likely give him so much more independence, so much more of a life in the community. Why shouldn't I give him that opportunity?

Because of the potential downside: so much of the success of shared living depended on the caregiver being the right match for the client. They would be sharing an apartment, as roommates. No others to cushion their interactions, no distractions—positive or negative. Would Nat get lonely? Would he have more opportunities to grow in terms of self-entertainment and self-care?

I knew right away who the caregiver had to be: John. He and Nat had been a great pairing from the start. John understood Nat's need for structure, downtime, and yet also new (but carefully explained, clearly laid out) experiences. Nat was comfortable with John's colorful personality.

I called him shortly after Nat's appointment. John was in, immediately. The salary was about the same, and in fact, the shared living stipend would be tax-free. John (and Nat) would have to move to a place for the two of them, because unlike a group home manager, he would be living with Nat. But moving was no obstacle—John didn't like his apartment at that time anyway. Now I had to be sure this was something Nat wanted.

I took him out for Starbucks a few days later. We settled into two armchairs, and while he was eating his chocolate chip cookie I started setting up the conversation, structuring the questions so that he would understand what I was asking him. To get Nat to answer anything, you have to ask him one way, and then reverse the order of the choice the next time, and then do it all over again, to be sure he is not simply taking the last choice out of default.

I wanted to be as certain as possible that a move like this was something Nat wanted, so I recorded our conversation. Here is the transcript:

I said, "I'm trying to figure out if Nat wants to live at Grove Street [the group home address] or at an apartment. Nat, do you want to live at Grove Street or an apartment?"

"A 'parment," Nat answered pretty quickly in his delightfully quirky way. He often combines words in ways that make sense even though they are technically grammatically incorrect: "Put some parmes on the spaghetti," or, "Grandpa Batch and GrandAnd" (Grandma Anne).

After he answered "a 'parment," I rephrased it: "Do you want to live in an apartment or Grove Street?" Nat understands "or."

"Live in an apartment." Ah, that was a pretty definite, confident response.

"Who are you going to live with?" I asked.

"Dana." Great! Now we had moved into actual content in our conversation. Dana is one of his housemates at the group home. (Dana did not come to live with Nat in the apartment. But I'm still hoping.)

And so, just about two years after Nat turned twenty-two, three living situations later, he was on his way to trying shared living. Nat was going to live in an apartment in a bustling fun neighborhood like where he'd grown up, which had been my vision at the very beginning. Unlike those early days, however, Nat's funding was already in place. The Department of Developmental Services supports shared living arrangements as a positive and preferable alternative to group homes because they are more "natural" than group homes—non-disabled living alongside disabled, building a life together.

The question that remained was, given that Dana was not going to live with them, would Nat be lonely living only with one other guy? Was Nat and John's relationship strong enough to support this dramatic change in lifestyle for Nat? Would Nat rise to the challenge of a less structured lifestyle?

Dr. Peter Gerhardt: teaching our guys what they need in the world

Ultimately, I have learned from Nat that anyone, autistic or not, will learn and grow if he is given the chance to try—though it won't necessarily be within his comfort zone. I have had this belief validated by one of my most cherished, knowledgeable experts: Dr. Peter Gerhardt. Peter is a world-renowned autism adulthood specialist, who for decades has been working with autistic people up and down the spectrum, helping them develop social skills in the working world and other areas of life. He is chair of the Scientific Council for the Organization for Autism Research.

I met Peter years ago, at a conference where we both presented, and his clarity and understanding of autism blew me away. That and his directness and honesty made me feel like I'd found a kindred spirit. Here I have included points from one of his online talks, and from conversations I've had with him, for the purpose of this chapter: to explain best practices in skill-building with autistic people.

If I could sum up Peter's philosophy, I think it would be that first and foremost, you need to teach skills that actually matter in a given autistic person's life, and not teach him superfluous skills that don't translate to what he needs to live as independently as possible. Second, in teaching these skills, you need to make sure there is a natural context in which the student can learn and then use them in the real world. This way you don't need to create artificial structures that don't exist outside the classroom. And finally, you need to teach by taking some risks—calculated risks, not crazy risks—keeping in mind, of course, that when you take risks you don't always succeed. To Peter, this should be okay. We all mess up sometimes. Why can't autistics be given the same leeway? Peter's answer: they should be. Peter sees the training of autistic people as part and parcel of retraining the world.

Peter's recommendations for someone with autism are all about being selective and canny about the skills you want to be acquired. Think about teaching in the proper context, think about taking healthy risks, and think about a more positive way to look at autism so that the rest of the world will, too.

Make sure the skill you teach is relevant

In one of his lectures, Peter said, "You have to think about what skills are most needed to help him succeed in the first place. What is the value of what you want to teach—why would he need the skill in the first place?"

Peter believes that we need to get out of the habit of teaching our guys just in black and white terms, or bad choice versus good choice. In real life there are so many choices. Frequently, when we teach kids on the spectrum, we teach them "either/or." This is too simplistic. We ask, "apple or banana?" They look at me to see what the right answer is. That's what they've been taught their entire life. It is a simplistic question because if I went up to you and asked if you wanted an apple or a banana, you would first look to see what kind of apple it was. Is it bruised, is it a Granny Smith? Do you want it whole, sliced with cheese? "You don't have a Granny Smith, well, I'll take a yellow." In other words, we can't be robotic ourselves when teaching any kind of skill, to any kind of person. We can't stop at either/or. We caregivers must under-stand the importance of choice-making in our guys' lives.

Another example Peter gives is tooth brushing, which is nor-mally a socially reinforced skill. But do the social rewards you and I get from brushing our teeth matter to an autistic person? If not, you might want to delay teaching this goal. He says, "You want to brush your teeth in the morning because you want to have fresh breath to talk to people or to get a kiss. But hygiene is not as immediately reinforced for autistic adults as it might be for me or you. We have to remember that someone with autism might not *want* to talk to people or get kissed, and therefore might not be motivated to brush his teeth." Therefore it is important to ask whether this autistic student actually needs this skill at this time. "We need to look at ways he can acquire skills that are of intrinsic value to him right now," Peter says. In other words, we cannot take it for granted that autistic people will automatically value skills that neurotypical people value.

Aim for the greatest efficiency of skill acquisition

Another factor in teaching autistic people a particular skill is to consider how easy it is to put that skill in place. How much energy do you want to devote to this effort? Is there a natural context in which to learn this skill? According to Peter, "Context is a critical variable as we try to teach this cohort of skills. For example, teachable moments—opportunities to respond—are important." Teaching color identification is the example Peter uses. "The best example is if we take John, a kid with classic ASD at age five, and we teach him color identification. 'Johnny touch red,' he touches red. 'Johnny touch blue,' he touches blue. He learns all sixty-four labels in the Crayola box. But—it took *one thousand* interactions. Some of us call that a skill," Gerhardt said with a touch of sarcasm, begging the question: what have we actually gained in all that effort?

Peter therefore recommends teaching skills that are possible to achieve in a reasonable amount of time and that make sense in the autistic person's real life. "Take the example of using a cell phone. A cell phone is a cheap and easy tool to acquire, and its uses are invaluable. It can teach kids to make and to receive calls," he said. "But there are also more subtle benefits: safety and independence.

They have to make sure their phone is with them at all times. This enables them to use a GPS to know where they are, and it also can help caregivers, employers, and parents to tell them where they are. Think of the kids who wander. Isn't it possible that if they always have a cell phone, they'd be able to tell someone how to find them? In the end, a simple cell phone can support great independence." This is the kind of skill that is a low-hanging fruit, in which the learning process is relatively simple to implement and that already exists naturally in our culture—implying that it is not rocket science to teach our guys, and that the right tasks might not require one thousand teachable moments.

Teach the right skills in the right context

Peter often speaks about how to build social skills naturally, to teach them in the environment where they are most likely to be used and where there are opportunities for feedback. Setting up skill-building in relevant surroundings, with built-in rewards, can lead to the highest degree of mastery.

Peter believes that too much rote learning inside a classroom—as in applied behavioral analysis programs—leads to skills that don't necessarily translate into the real world. He said, "My bottom line is that each student needs to be able to transfer control to the actual environment." The skills we teach must be learned in the appropriate environment, and we must be sure that they are relevant to the student's actual life. "I'm much more interested in how context works with altering the student's behavior," Peter says.

Peter also has no patience for excessive emphasis on "appropriate" behavior over common sense (appropriate in quotes because I feel that the word is used pejoratively with autism; some of the so-called inappropriate or undesirable autistic behavior is essential to the autistic person to help him stay calm or organize his thoughts). He even advocates a messier outcome if that's what it takes to teach the more important skill. "We need to look at what he's doing in the community—how independent is he?"

Consider risk as an aid to independence

We need to have a bigger expectation of what our guys can do. We neurotypical people put more limits on those with ASD than is necessary. Peter urges us to always ask, "Why *can't* he do this? . . . If we start to proceed in that direction, no doubt we'll fail sometimes. But we need to come to grips with the concept of risk. What is an acceptable level of risk? People [of all sorts] die in accidents in home all the time. Risk is with us *all* the time. There's no life in which there are zero risks.

"We all make mistakes," Peter says. "An Aspie I knew punched his roommate when he found out he'd had sex with the girl he liked. Of course, no one should do that. And most of the time we don't. We have such a high standard for guys on the spectrum. 'Oh, that's aggression!' we say. When he punches someone is it a crisis? Life isn't perfect." There is a strong undercurrent of confidence Peter has in his autistic students, a healthy openness to their abilities to land on their feet.

Like Peter, I feel that the symbiosis of my attitude with Nat's is necessary to his success. Sometimes Ned and I say with wonder, "I think he really knows when people are on his side." But this shouldn't be such a revelation. We need to remember that of course he knows! Why wouldn't he know? His perception, his sensitivity to what's in the air should never be questioned. If anything, he feels too much and it gets in his way. So we ought to begin with the understanding that our autistic loved one wants to be with—and does much better with—people who get him. People who like him. If our starting point is an eagerness to see how he can soar, I believe that he will already be halfway there.

Gerhardt emphasizes that we are all too quick to limit autistic people in what they can do. "People with autism are just people.

In realistic terms, I am competent in what I do. Try to force me to be an accountant, and I am going to be a complete and utter failure." In his experience, "25 percent of the community is very open and very eager to engage with autistic people. They want to help. Another 50 percent of the public is nervous but open. They don't want something to be screwed up, they don't want any mistakes in the workplace. And the last 25 percent of the general public are untrainable. I don't have time to deal with them," he says. "Work with the other 75 percent." Social competence is not just a one-way street. "It is up to *other* people to be more flexible. Let's start talking about how *typical* people can respond." Peter believes that the non-autistic world can and should change, just as much as autistic people should. Interpersonal contact is the most effective way to teach social skills. Much like what UCSB's Dr. Lynn Koegel has found in her autism research, Peter asserts that neurotypical people need to continue to be exposed to different types of minds.

Peter feels that, perhaps most of all, we need to change the way we talk about autism. "We only talk about the downside, about the negative. We say, 'Autism is a horrible developmental disability, it is expensive, we need to research it, we need to cure it.' Then we come along and say, 'He can work for you.' If you think about it, these are two very different messages. It is no wonder the public is confused about and even intolerant of autism."

Navigating social norms

I interviewed some families to try to get an idea of what particular struggles have come up for their autistic loved ones, other than those strictly related to creating housing or day occupations. Some families are overwhelmed by keeping all of the advocacy going, trying to keep their funding organized and at adequate levels. Some are dealing with relationships and sexuality, some with desire for independence. What follows are individual stories about challenges and their resolutions, or the lessons learned.

I talked to Susan, an autism mom whose son Paul is Nat's age. His autism manifests itself in depression and sensory issues, as well as in difficulty combing through social situations. This last challenge is possibly Paul's toughest, because it has so far kept him from living a life he wants: one with independence, and a girlfriend.

Paul is the oldest of six. As a child, Paul was verbal and affectionate. On the one hand he was very passive and on the other very sensitive. The sound of a new heater in their house would set him off. If he was watching a video and static interfered, he'd claw at his face.

At one point Susan sent him to a preschool, but they had just one car so it was difficult. Eventually, she decided that she could be his preschool—because she was actually already doing it. "We were very hands on, working Play-Doh, coloring, digging in the dirt." Ultimately, she didn't send any of her kids to preschool, since they had a big family and she realized that the window of time with little ones is short. "And once they start kindergarten," she said, "it's six hours out of the day." Susan ended up homeschooling Paul. Being very religious, she chose a Mennonite curriculum. It was black and white, simple, not overly stimulating, and uncluttered. Susan was largely satisfied with this educational program, but by the time they'd gone through the entire curriculum, Paul was still not reading. Susan said, "We had moved, and there were a lot of changes. I was pregnant with our fifth child, my husband worked long hours, and Paul reacted by playing with his feces and urinating behind furniture. He was speaking in echolalia . . . it was just really hard, very hard."

They sent Paul to kindergarten at a private school. He seemed fine, but by the end of the year the school said they could not graduate him to first grade because they believed he had a severe learning disability.

The Portsmouth, Virginia, public school district had an excellent program for people with autism. By the time Paul was almost eight, he went to first grade with his brother, who was two years younger, and the notes started coming home from his teacher on the first day: "I can't reach him." But then, after psychological evaluation, they put him in a classroom with four other kids. He sat in a cubicle facing the wall. He wasn't distracted. He learned to read.

At twenty, in 2010, he finished special education classes in high school and joined his younger brother in walking across the stage on graduation day. That marked his transition into adulthood. He worked very hard at his dad's warehouse, but it was difficult, as he was moody and lonely. During his darkest moments, Susan has turned to her deep belief in God and the solace of religious ritual and faith. At one particularly difficult time with Paul, Susan said, when he had punched a hole in a wall out of frustration, "We were in New York for a trade show and he called me at 4:30 a.m." She prayed with him via cell phone and described its calming effect: "Contemplative prayer is a tool for someone with an autistic teenager, similar to bracing their arms in a hug; especially since I couldn't be there to calm him down."

Paul attended a program at the University of North Carolina, Greensboro, which has a tiered system of support for special needs students. "They are classified as UNCG students but they have a curriculum geared toward life skills," Susan explained. "They walk at graduation, and though they don't receive a diploma, they can earn a certificate in Community Integrative Studies. The age range is wide. A fifty-five-year-old student with Down syndrome graduated and opened up a book store on the beach near her parents." Success like this made Susan very hopeful for Paul, but at that time in his life, the college-away-from-home experience was not meant to be.

Even with the support of the UNCG system—a program called Beyond Academics—things did not go smoothly for Paul. People on the spectrum who attend college may slip through the cracks, because the kind of support they need is perhaps less tangible than for those with other developmental disabilities or with cognitive delays. One link in the chain of support can make the difference between a successful college experience or a disastrous one.

While attending UNCG, Paul lived in his own apartment, where he had someone looking in on him twenty-five hours a week. They took him grocery shopping and helped him get organized. Paul is very athletic, and he joined a running club. He biked, lifted weights, swam with a club, and even played on the UNCG ultimate frisbee team.

However, he had three meltdowns within that two-year period. "His socialization was stunted and he resisted the social opportunities with other Beyond Academics students," Susan said. "He's a bit of a snob. He doesn't want to be associated with other people with disabilities. That's where I struggle between high functioning and low functioning. When he's depressed and stubborn, it's difficult to help him. To me, that's low functioning."

Susan's feelings about, the seemingly arbitrary designations we give to people on the vast autism spectrum are similar to mine. None of the categorizations feel legitimate. Autistic people can be all over the map in terms of functioning. I understood this to be what the term "splinter skills" means, something I learned about years ago when Nat was first diagnosed. "Paul can do a lot, but he needs a lot of support. And there's also a lot he can't do. A homeless person once talked him out of his money. He's in a difficult spot as far as his future is concerned," Susan said. "It's like he's outside of a glass window. He sees what he wants but he can't get it. He developed an obsession with having a girlfriend. He'd meet [a girl], get her phone number, and call her ten times in a row—or knock on the door until she'd answer. He said to her, 'You don't know how great I am. You need to be my friend, then marry me, then have my son.'"

Susan told me that, of course, this girl was "freaked out." In turn, Paul wandered around his apartment complex, furious. "He went to a streetlamp and yanked it off its base—out of the cement. Then he went over to a picnic table and pulled off two planks." Another time, Paul got so upset about something that he tried to step off a moving bus. Later on in our conversation, Susan told me sadly, "I'd bought him a parakeet, I'd go visit him . . . it was so sad because this parakeet symbolized my son. Quiet, alone. It had the same feeling as Paul's apartment, the feeling of loneliness."

Sadly for our guys on the spectrum, there is not much public tolerance for people with challenges like Paul's. Behaviors like Paul's make some in society wary of those on the spectrum, unsure how far they'll go with their obsessions, or whether their outbursts are just a way of expressing inner frustration.

After that incident, when Susan went and picked him up, she told him that he needed a break, and he was surprised. "I do?" he asked her. Before leaving Greensboro for the last time, in a waiting room at the psychiatrist's office, in broad daylight, he laid his head on her lap and napped before his appointment. He was twenty-two at the time. Susan felt like crying.

Although Susan didn't send Paul back to college, she did not let him founder. At home, he took a computer class and then a drawing class at the community college, and he's currently taking piano lessons. He also has a dog. "I don't know what the future is for my son," Susan said, but as she told her daughter and her husband, "So what? He makes weird noises, but at least he's not drinking, or on the internet with pornography. He cooks, does his own laundry, and takes care of his dog."

Paul does have job responsibilities. He works assembling games for the family's company, Cactus Game Design, which uses popular secular games like Apples to Apples, Scrabble, and Cranium, and creates Bible editions. "We have a game called Redemption; the appeal is not only sophisticated game play, but collecting. Paul assembles these card packs. Watching him is like witnessing a well-oiled machine," Susan said.

Now Paul lives in Susan's basement, while her daughters occupy the third floor. "We can't be more than thirty minutes away from him at any point. He has it pretty good here, but it's a little lonesome, too. We live in the sticks. He talked about moving to a town about an hour away, and buying a house. It was scary to have to tell him, 'No Paul, we're sorry, you're not doing that. It's not safe, you don't drive, how would you get around, where would you work?' Surprisingly, he consented with, 'OK.'"

Susan has hope, because anything good may happen. That is her faith talking. If things don't change, Susan says, "When we get old and feeble, one of his siblings will take over. He is maturing, being more pleasant, not so manic. Recently he was having a mood, and I just talked him out of it. I was here, and I'm glad for that. This is how we live. We don't know what the future holds for Paul, but we're all here for each other."

Being autistic, gay, and coming out

Donna's son Carson will be twenty-three in in the spring. Out of respect for the family's privacy, I have changed their names. "Because Carson can't speak for himself," Donna explained.

In Canada, adult services begin at nineteen. Carson didn't get a diploma; upon finishing school, he went to an adult autism day program, and he's been out of that for a year. We wanted him to work, to have more physical fitness activity in his day; to learn more about nutrition, and independent living skills. It was a small program, eight students, on a range of the spectrum. They did some fitness, some vocational training, but he wasn't progressing well. I think he was bored—a lot of behaviors were coming out. We had consultants go in and observe, but we ultimately took him out of the program.

Carson has a job, two hours twice a week. "He cleans a theater, washes the washrooms, and loves to vacuum and dust. He has an employment coach. Now they are trying to increase the hours at that job, or if there are no more hours available, maybe elsewhere." He also does tae kwon do on Saturdays with a friend, a young man from his former day program. "They do stuff afterward—hiking, outdoors lunch. Both peers have a staff person with them. This friend also has a job, does the same kind of things Carson does: fitness every day, learning healthy nutrition, journaling, spin class," Donna said, illustrating how fulfilling our guys' lives can be.

When Carson got his theater job, he apparently asked Donna if this meant that he would be acting on a stage. "He loves drama and theater, likes retro stuff," said Donna. "He was already a Disney kid, and he knew a lot of dialogue he would use appropriately. At a Starbucks he said, 'Hold on Sugar, Daddy's got a sweet tooth tonight.' Once he said 'Hello Legs' to an attractive girl with long legs. He has a lot of insight into others, but not his own situation."

Then, in the last year or so, Carson began to have episodes acting out scenes and sometimes things became dangerous, such as when he would run away or interact with strangers. Donna talked to a doctor who saw him frequently, and at the time the doctor thought that Carson's challenging behavior and acting out was related to Donna's daughter's approaching wedding. But then, at a more recent appointment, the doctor had a new thought: he suggested that Carson might be gay. "Carson is obsessed with young men," said Donna. "He's always had crushes on men, friends of my daughter who are men. But he also really liked Drew Barrymore and Winona Ryder." She added, "My husband and I each have a gay brother; there are lots of gay people in the family."

So Donna and her husband tried to teach Carson what they thought he needed to know about gay sexuality, relationships, and personal safety. "Carson said, 'Oh, straight is the opposite of gay.'" Donna then named a bunch of family members and he identified who was straight or gay. She then asked him about himself and he said, "Gay."

But Donna is still not certain of his understanding of being gay. She told me: "A day or two after our conversation about family members, he'd said of his coworker, 'Rob is special, I'm attracted to him, I have a crush on him.'" This was a new sort of language for Carson, and he seemed embarrassed when Donna pursued the conversation and asked him, "Is Rob straight or gay?" Donna had never seen him embarrassed before then. This really meant something to Donna—it was as if Carson *was* truly aware of his feelings, of homosexuality, and of Rob, the coworker.

Donna tried to figure out how this epiphany had come to be. One thing she realized was that around that time, Carson had watched a film called *American Wedding*, where someone in the movie said, "I'm attracted to you, you're special." Those, of course, were the exact words he'd used for Rob. She said, "When he told Rob he was special, Rob had said, 'you're special, too.'"

All of this articulation of emotion was in a very natural, comfortable manner. I am reluctant to use the phrase "normal and appropriate" here, because what is normal for Carson is not the same as for Donna or me. Why can't there be two different normals? Or more? I believe they can all coexist. What Donna and I are interested in is helping our sons live fulfilling lives—whatever that may mean—and be as comfortable with themselves as possible. Like any of us, Carson and Nat do have to learn to be a constructive part of society, but there is a line between functioning comfortably enough and forcing oneself to change for others.

Donna's goal now is to further identify Carson's preferences, help him live happily in that identity, and make healthy choices. "I don't think he will ever have sex. He doesn't even really masturbate. We had a sexuality educator; she developed a book on how to masturbate, but we haven't had any evidence that he does. It could be the meds he's on," Donna said. They looked for help for Carson, and took some recommendations from Dr. Peter Gerhardt. She started a sexual health program with Carson. "However, we talked about sex only from a straight perspective, not a gay one," Donna said, reminding me once again how recent Carson's discovery is. "He does know what heterosexual sex is. He said to me, 'The man puts his hard penis into the woman's soft vagina.' But I don't know if he knows what men do together."

Donna feels that if Carson were not autistic he would be totally out-of-the-closet gay. "We're on the lookout for signs, and how to make him at ease with it. I really do think he has some insight into what it is to be gay." Donna, in her typical forthright way, said, "He loves to get mani-pedis, and he picks colors he's seen on Katy Perry and Johnny Depp. He chose to wear Tiffany blue nail polish for my daughter's wedding." Because of their shared passion for going to nail salons, Donna and Carson have a fun activity they can do together. Another one of Carson's favorite days of the year is the Pride Parade. "He loves it," Donna said, "he's involved with it; he's on the water truck every year. They shoot big water cannons at the people parading. It's a family event, and we go down in our rainbow clothes. My sister and I hold hands, the dykes on bikes, pretending we're lesbians." Clearly humor and acceptance are big parts of Donna's family.

I believe that Donna and Carson's openness to each other's interests is a key part of their successful relationship. I, too, am always on the lookout for mutual interests with Nat so that we can do things together. But then again, I don't know that he wants to do more things with me. He seems happiest when he is going off to social group activities or the Special Olympics practices and events—with peers. Here, too, is a dividing line that must be respected. He has very different social needs from me—and that should be OK. I still have to get used to that sometimes, though.

The attitude of tolerance and acceptance found in Donna's family isn't universal; if he had been born into a different family, Donna acknowledges, "Carson could have been excommunicated or something like that." But this would never happen in Donna's family. "It's just who he is. I'm so proud to have these kids. I'm so proud to be their mother. And his father is a gentle, supportive, good man." They are invested in each other, they love each other, and that is the bottom line. Carson will have a safe and secure future because Donna has worked out a very protective setup with her daughter. When the time comes, she said, "My daughter and her husband are in the will; they'll take over his care."

Nat and the girl on the T

By the time Nat was in his twenties, I had pretty much stopped thinking about him having sophisticated or romantic relationships. For a long time, he had seemed so content with just hanging out on the edges of groups, being on teams, or going with his social group to the theater, out to dinner, or to see the Red Sox.

But something was in the air during the early spring of his twenty-fifth year. I think it got into my head from talking to a friend during Special Olympics basketball practice. She was telling me about how her son, who was nineteen and had higher verbal skills than Nat, seemed to be looking at girls quite a bit. "I don't know, maybe there's some girl that would . . ." She didn't finish her thought, but I knew what she was going to say.

"Yeah, I think about that for Nat all the time," I said, "but I don't think it's in the cards."

She looked at me with a frown. "Why not?"

Why not? Well, couldn't she see that he could not converse with people, much less chat up a young woman? How would that happen? I do not know the first thing about teaching him to approach a woman and begin a connection with her.

But the more I thought about it, the more my friend's words stung. How could I close the door on this very momentous part of life for my beloved son? Without even trying?

But hadn't I tried? I had wanted to arrange a night at the movies for Nat and a younger girl on his basketball team, who had shown a little interest in him. She had messaged him a few times on Facebook. They had had a tiny conversation, which was huge for Nat.

I'd written to her father, offering to stay with them in the theater, but in a different row. A few days later came the response: "She doesn't want to." Ugh, my heart burned from that one. And I had no idea what Nat thought about it, but I'm sure he remembered talking about the possibility with me—Nat doesn't forget anything.

John, Nat's wonderful caregiver, had succeeded in teaching Nat appropriate responses to some-small talk kinds of interactions. Now when our younger son, Max, comes home for a visit, he'll say, "Hey Nat, what's up," and Nat will answer, "Not much." So I wondered if John could teach him some kind of brief give-and-take with a girl, something like, "Hey, how's it going?" And after she answers, he says, "Well, gotta go." A friendly beginning. But John just laughed nervously and said, "Oh, man, I'm not going to go there with Nat!" So I didn't know if I could push it.

Then came the Sunday on the T. Nat, my husband, Ned, and I were coming back from a trip downtown. The train wasn't too crowded. There was a seat open, next to a young woman with long, curly brown hair, probably in her early twenties. She noticed Nat, and seemed to become more self-conscious—I don't know how I knew that, exactly, but it was as if she had pulled her body together a little more sharply, somehow, a little more there.

And so had Nat. He was leaning forward, his eyes were their clearest blue, refreshing like water. I said nothing to him; I pretended I wasn't with him. I kept talking to Ned, who was standing leaning on the pole, facing Nat. "Is he sucking his thumb?" I whispered through my teeth.

"No," said Ned.

"Silly talk? Flapping?"

"Nope."

This was singular. Nat *always* stimmed on the T. But this was not always. This time was different: he was next to a pretty girl, who was aware of him. And every time I caught his eye, he looked straight into mine, crisp consciousness sketching his irises. Nat was on.

Eventually the girl started gathering her stuff to get off. It seemed like Nat was not aware that he would have to let her out.

She stood up and mumbled, "Excuse me," and I was about to intervene—of course—but something held me back. Why not let him figure this out?

And he did. He half-stood and let her out.

That's it. Nothing had happened. And yet—perhaps something had.

Things to Consider About Loving and Supporting People on the Spectrum

- Think of difference rather than deficit; unique rather than abnormal. Make sure you are not pounding a polyhedron into a round hole. Presume competence.
- Be prepared for any possibility. It may not be what you think. Be open. Focus on acceptance rather than eradication of differences.
- Check up on your professionals: staff, teachers, physicians, and therapists. Be sure they are not conveying judgmental, harsh, or destructive messages to your autistic loved one. Life is hard enough!

Resources for Relationships, Sexuality, and Autism

- iAssist Communicator is one of the only communication apps I could find specifically for adults. The site boasts a "sleek, mature design," and is "specifically focused on the more cognitively challenged. The founder is a psychologist and a mom with an adult with autism. With the unique needs of these individuals in mind, the app incorporates photos rather than more abstract drawings, larger images, and functional language." Dr. Peter Gerhardt is also on the management team at iAssist, so that in itself is a great recommendation: www.iassistcompany.com

- Capitalize on obsessions and rituals as a starting point to connection. Applied behavioral analysis (ABA) and other behavioral modifications can teach certain pragmatics that will help foster higher-functioning skills of every sort, as well as independence. Also, utilize the relational therapies that begin with the autistic person's preferences and hobbies and build skills outward from specific interests, like Pivotal Response Therapy (PRT) (www.autismprthelp.com/) and Developmental, Individual Difference, Relationship-based (DIR): www.icdl.com/DIR.
- ACT Programs from the Governor's Council of Minnesota are all about self-advocacy skills and knowing your rights as a person with a disability trying to function in the world, particularly on the job: www.selfadvocacy.org/programs/work-skills.htm
- The organization AASPIRE has a handy resource, the AASPIRE Healthcare Toolkit: Primary Care Resources for Adults on the Autism Spectrum and their Primary Care Providers (autismandhealth.org)
- Healthy Transitions, Moving from Pediatric to Adult Health Care, New York State Institute for Health Transition Training: www.healthytransitionsny.org. This website is for youth with developmental disabilities ages fourteen to twenty-five, family caregivers, service coordinators, and health-care providers.
- Speak it! is an app that allows you to select text and it will read it aloud to you: www.chrome.google.com/webstore/detail/speakit
- Students with autism interested in pursuing post-secondary education can apply for $3,000 scholarships through OAR: www.ow.ly/HMkaN

- Between the Lines Advanced (for Adults) is an app that allows the user to work on understanding subtlety and nuance in communication: itunes.apple.com/us/app/between-the-lines-advanced-hd/id574685561?mt=8
- Job interview coaching software: www.jobinterviewtraining.net
- The Autism Research Institute has a lot of material about autism adulthood sexual and social issues: www.autism.com/news_agi_ebulletin
- BCCH (British Columbia, Canada Children's Hospital) website: http://www.bcchildrens.ca/our-services/support-services/transition-to-adult-care/youth-toolkit/sexual-health
- Attend the TASH (originally stood for The Association for Persons with Severe Handicaps) Conferences, tash.org,which are all about inclusion and skill-building. They are for self-advocates, family members, professionals, and autism friends. Find your region and see what training they can offer you.
- Jess Wilson's blog *Diary of a Mom* for a great example of a loving, smart-as-a-whip perspective of autism acceptance: adiaryofamom.com/

Books and Articles

- Stephen Shore's classic book *Beyond the Wall: Personal Experiences with Autism and Asperger's Syndrome* gives insight into living on the Spectrum. (Autism Asperger Publishing Company, 2003)
- Chantal Sicile-Kira, advocate, speaker, author, and mother of Jeremy, a very accomplished young man with autism,

wrote *A Full Life With Autism: From Learning to Forming Relationships to Independence* to convey the possibility and potential of those with autism (St. Martin's, 2012).

- *Sexuality and Safety with Tom and Ellie* book series, by Kate E. Reynolds, Jonathon Powell (Jessica Kingsley, 2014).
- Check out *Life, Animated* by Ron Suskind for an in-depth description of how he utilized Affinity Therapy (similar to PRT and DIR) to help his own autistic son become more social and connected to others (Kingswell, 2014).
- *A Regular Guy: Growing Up with Autism*, author and autism mom Laura Shumaker's remarkable, honest, and poignant book about her adult son Matthew's emergence into happy adulthood (Landscape, 2008).
- *Born on a Blue Day*, by Daniel Tammet, is an insightful perspective on being gay and having Asperger's (Freepress, 2007).
- "How to Work with Someone with Autism," article in MarketWatch by Brent Betit and Dorie Clark (http://www.marketwatch.com/story/how-to-work-with-someone-with-autism-2015-02-11).
- *Life and Love: Positive Strategies for Autistic Adults*, by Zosia Zaks (Autism Asperger Publishing Company, 2006).
- *Growing Up on the Spectrum: A Guide to Life, Love, and Learning for Teens and Young Adults with Autism and Asperger's*, by Claire S. LaZebnik (Penguin, 2009).
- *Decoding Dating: A Guide to the Unwritten Social Rules of Dating for Men With Asperger Syndrome (Autism Spectrum Disorder)*, by John Miller (Jessica Kingsley, 2014).
- *Autism and Its Medical Management*, by Michael Chez MD (Jessica Kingsley, 2009).
- *Living Well on the Spectrum: How to Use Your Strengths to Meet the Challenges of Asperger Syndrome/High-Functioning Autism*, by Valerie L. Gaus, PhD (Guilford Press, 2007).

- *Living Independently on the Autism Spectrum: What You Need to Know to Move into a Place of Your Own, Succeed at Work, Start a Relationship, Stay Safe, and Enjoy Life as an Adult on the Autism Spectrum,* by Lynne Soraya (Adams Media, 2013).
- For a new perspective on gender and sexuality, check out Jennifer Boylan's book, *She's Not There* (Broadway Books, 2013).

CHAPTER SIX

THE STRUGGLES OF APPARENTLY HIGH-FUNCTIONING AUTISTIC ADULTS

Trying to connect with people my age
Attempting to reveal my unique vision
But ending up alone and unengaged
Feeling like my life needs a total revision
Just a normal day
Can't You See
Can't you see
I just want to have a friend
Can't you see
I need the same connections in the end

—Scott Lentine, "Just a Normal Day"

ALL OF NAT'S LIFE, I have experienced what I call "Asperger's envy." I envied the dad in my earliest support group, whose little daughter could play with toys the way they were intended by Mattel, and I envied Dr. Spock, the friend whose kid could not talk when Nat could, who seemed so very autistic, but who then as a teen went on to be able to travel anywhere on his own. I was always jealous of the ones who were included in the public schools, who weren't sent half an hour away to a special autism school as Nat was.

I am not proud of this, but the truth is that I do get jealous of high-functioning autistic adults, the ones who might even self-diagnose late in life. Those who say, "Ah, now I understand why things have been so hard for me all my life, why I was awkward, bullied, why I never fit in. I am autistic!" And yet one particular friend, a former Wall Street wizard, was saying just this, fluently and fluidly, sitting in a coffee shop in his suit and tie. I had to make a real effort not to dismiss him. What are we supposed to make of the adult who says he is autistic but seems light-years away from our own autistic child? How is it that Temple Grandin, who is fully verbal and able to navigate cities, airports, and conferences, has the same diagnosis as Nat? According to the American Psychiatric Association's Diagnostic and Statistical Manual V, the autism spectrum is very, very broad:

People with ASD tend to have communication deficits, such as responding inappropriately in conversations, misreading nonverbal interactions, or having difficulty building friendships appropriate to their age. In addition, people with ASD may be overly dependent on routines, highly sensitive to changes in their environment, or intensely focused on inappropriate items. Again, the symptoms of people with ASD will fall on a continuum, with some individuals showing mild symptoms and others having much more severe symptoms.

The autism spectrum is even broader than in Nat's early days, when we had on one end classic infantile autism, PDD, PDD-NOS, high-functioning autism, and Asperger's. Now it is so broad that there are scarcely any terms at all. Asperger's is not separate. Even the term "high-functioning autism" is a misnomer. HFA is a term that makes you think that this person has "autism lite." In reality, there are very difficult social issues that each person must parse, or terribly acute sensory problems, all of which may lead to incapacitation of one kind or another. If HFA is code for "verbal," then we should say "verbal." Being nonverbal, however, and being able to type, may make someone previously thought to be low functioning now appear high.

As autism-enlightened as I am, it is still very hard for me to believe that some people who seem so "normal" indeed have autism. They can answer questions in a crowded coffee shop, they get my jokes, they look me in the eye ! They aren't flapping, they aren't rocking. How is this the same disorder as Nat's autism?

And yet it is.

I know that autism is different in every person: if you've met one autistic person, you've met one autistic person. We can't compare people in this way, and to do so is unproductive and narrow-minded. Autism has so many characteristics and co-occurring disorders like intellectual disability, expressive language impairment, or sensory integration difficulties. I constantly have to bear this in mind when talking to people with autism. You don't have to be like Nat to be autistic; being verbal and academically skilled does not imply an easy life. In fact, sometimes I think Nat may be happier than someone with higher verbal and academic skills because of how much more challenging it is to need to function directly in the world, supporting yourself (for lack of services) and trying to have friends. There is so little understanding (and I have proven that here with my own prejudices) of the verbally savvy autistic that life among the neurotypical may be a terrible hardship at times—as it is indeed for my Wall Street friend.

Autism is a very broad spectrum, as we all know by now, and the way someone gets to be "on it" is if they have a few of the many characteristics/deficits associated with ASD: difficult/different social interaction; rote, routine, rigid requirements; sensory sensitivities; processing problems or unusual ways of taking in information; eccentric behavioral outlets.

Many of these adults on the spectrum stepped forward to talk to me when I started this book, and I am so grateful for the window they opened into my cloudy ideas about the spectrum. Their stories will give you an idea of the particular, specific struggles of so-called "high-functioning" and "low-functioning" autism, and the kind of success some autistics have nevertheless had in their lives.

Autism and self-discovery through writing

Scott Lentine is a friend on the spectrum living in Massachusetts. We spoke briefly, but Scott has a much easier time expressing his thoughts in writing than verbally, so he emailed me some of his thoughts.

I chose to interview Scott as an example of someone with autism who struggles and yet has created a meaningful life for himself. But Scott believes that his success began with a wise and understanding family. He feels that the single strongest factor in his own competence in the world is the way his parents understood his needs; particularly his need to know about himself and his disability. "Parents should tell their child about their disability by the time they are in preschool or elementary school," Scott wrote. He pointed out that there are ample signs of disability, and Scott feels that a parent owes it to their child to pay attention to them and take action. "The parent can tell if the child has a disability if the child's speech patterns are lagging behind the norm, if the child has troubling making normal eye contact, if certain sensations frighten the child, if he or she has trouble reading or writing, and/or seems unaware of their surroundings," Scott explained.

Scott realized he had a disability during elementary school. "I was nonverbal until a little over five years old. Of course, I knew I was different, but there was nothing I could do about the disability," he wrote. His self-awareness even at such an early age illustrates how you just cannot generalize about people with autism, and that you should not subscribe to the stereotypes out there.

Scott's satisfying adulthood may have been a result of a few key educators during his school years. During both elementary and middle school, Scott had devoted special education teachers who knew the challenges of autism and had good strategies. The school psychologist was also an excellent resource, which is not always the case, particularly when school systems cut supports like psychologists and social workers. So often I have found that it is in middle school, during those crucial and potentially excruciating years, that our guys slip through the cracks. Scott was lucky to have had supports all along the way.

"In high school, I had a resource room as a study period to ask questions about homework or finish up on tests. I had accommodations like extra time on exams, use of a note taker, and being seated in the front of the room." Because of these accommodations, Scott was mainstreamed in all courses during high school. "I was a member of National Honor Society and did some statistical and score-keeping work for the volleyball and basketball teams," he said.

Scott went to Merrimack College in North Andover, graduating in 2010. His college experience was overall a positive one. However, life at Merrimack was not easy for him. "In many ways, I felt like a fish out of water when I started my collegiate years at Merrimack. I had to rely on students and an ADA form from my advisor to help facilitate the note-taking processes in the classroom. At the same time, I did make some new friends at Merrimack. From making social connections, I got involved in service learning programs at elementary schools in nearby Lawrence. There, I helped some students from lower socioeconomic backgrounds improve their mathematic and science skills through a STEM (Science, Technology, Engineering, and Math) program." A Federal education program, STEM is devoted to improving the experience of undergraduate students in math and science; to "better serving groups historically underrepresented in STEM fields; and designing graduate education for tomorrow's STEM workforce." (www.ed.gov/stem)

In his senior year of high school, Scott tried to do as much of the typical college thing as everyone else. "I applied to a good number of schools. I went through the same method of applications as anyone else," he said. Ultimately, he chose Merrimack because it was close to his family—he could be a commuter, living at home. Merrimack also had small classes of twenty to twenty-five students, and its disability services were enough to keep him going. These included extra time on exams, and receiving notes from professors and other students. "Overall, for the first couple of years, it could have been better mainly if there had been professional notetakers," Scott said. "Note-taking can be difficult; I have trouble catching up at times if the professor is a really fast talker. I believe my ADA advisors were not as experienced with people on the autism spectrum as they should have been. . . . I think the disability services a college offers is key," he told me. He was emphatic that people with autism who apply to college must make sure that the disability services offered are adequate. Colleges, for their part, should utilize ADA advisors and professors who have tremendous experience with people on the spectrum.

Scott started writing poetry over three years ago. His motivation sprang from a need to express his own experiences, wishes, and thought processes about autistic life. "I discovered there weren't that many songs or poems about autism." His ability to write poems filled this void for him, and his skill grew over time. Over the past years, Scott's poems have received positive receptions from many in the autism and general communities, including a radio interview with an NPR journalist.

Scott now works for the Arc of Massachusetts, which he credits in part to a wonderful job coach. He had to research supports to find this job coach using his own resources because he did not qualify for much public funding—unlike Nat, who receives funding for a part-time job coach.

Despite the enormous struggles people with Asperger's encounter, it is often unlikely that they will have any significant funding because of their normal to high IQs. In many states, funding for people with autism is still decided based on "intelligence" rather than functioning levels, and plenty of people who have high IQs desperately need supports for work, navigating the community, and organization. In Massachusetts this is about to change because of the passage of the Autism Omnibus Bill, which removes IQ from the equation. The Massachusetts Advocates for Children reports that there will be an "extension of Department of Developmental Services (DDS) eligibility to many persons with autism, Prader-Willi Syndrome, and Smith-Magenis Syndrome." (www.massadvocates.org/mac-victory-autism-omnibus-bill)

Hopefully other states will follow, and then we have to hope that along with the legislation, there will be funds appropriated to implement it.

Through the Autism-Asperger's Association of New England (AANE), Scott discovered the LifeMAP (Life Management Assistance Program) program, which led to finding his life coach. The AANE website describes LifeMAP as follows:

> LifeMAP provides practical assistance to individuals with Asperger Syndrome (AS) and related conditions. LifeMAP provides intensive, highly individualized coaching by professionals with expertise in both AS and specific content areas. Coaches focus on identifying and overcoming the specific barriers each client faces so that the clients can increase their levels of independence towards reaching their full potential. (www.lifemap.aane.org)

Scott attributed much of his job competence to LifeMAP:

> *I received most of my job training from my life coach. He has helped me focus on creating a resume and cover letter, finding jobs on websites like Indeed, Craigslist, and Career Builder, and continuing to build on social resources. At the Arc, I work as an administrative assistant/public policy intern. My duties include persuading legislators via email to improve health care, employment, and educational resources for people with developmental*

disabilities in the Commonwealth, editing databases in Excel, doing thank you letters and envelopes for Arc donors, and answering the phone.

Scott also does active advocacy, visiting the Massachusetts State House to persuade legislators to utilize resources for disabled citizens. "I have been there for three years and have supports from my boss and fellow coworkers, as well as fellow student interns from Brandeis," he wrote, reminding me that a good workplace must have built-in supports—colleagues who understand how to accommodate autism.

Aside from the poetry, Scott has hobbies and tries to keep his family and other social connections strong. "My favorite thing about myself is that I have a tremendous ability to retain a lot of information that I have used over the past years of my life. I also have good relationships with my family members and numerous friends. I am very friendly towards pretty much all people that I meet. I love dogs, traveling, going to concerts, spending time at my summer house in Marshfield, visiting my older brother in Boston on weekends, staying in shape, reading, hanging out with friends, and meeting new people."

Scott's Wisdom and Advice on Autism Adulthood

- When exploring suitable colleges, look online to see the autism support services offered there.
- Look into colleges that offer STEM programs.
- Apply to several schools. Contact the people in disability services and find out specifics about the kind of help they have. Not all disability services are alike!
- Utilize the skills of a job coach or life coach to maneuver the social subtleties of the workplace.

- Find an Autism-Asperger's support network, either nearby or online. The resources and common bonds are invaluable.
- For parents and caregivers, it is important to know what each individual's talents are, and to understand that not everybody can learn the same way.

Freeing oneself from a legacy of domestic abuse

I had gotten to know Dusya from various autism self-advocacy get-togethers. We met for this interview over coffee in Cambridge, Massachusetts, and we talked for about an hour. Dusya is a young woman diagnosed at the Asperger's end of the spectrum. At the time of the interview, she had no front teeth; she explained to me that she was in the middle of a big dental procedure that her father had refused her when she was growing up. (Months later I saw her beautiful new smile.) She is recently married, but is living with a roommate in Boston until she and her husband figure out how to find the right place for them. "Four years ago I moved with my mother to the South End . . . We moved to Boston to kind of start a new life."

Even though she's had a hard life, Dusya is not one to seek pity. She is an autism activist, a board member of Autistic Self-Advocacy Network (ASAN), a national group that lobbies legislators, corporations, and the media to change the treatment and perception of people with autism, and to improve policies around autism rights. Dusya's issues are less about the services and supports she needs, and more about the injustices that occur in autistics' lives based on the public not understanding. "Everyone's aware!" she said. "It's *understanding* that's needed."

Even though Dusya herself does not typically encounter mistreatment out in the world, she understands cruelty and ignorance firsthand. She had a very oppressive father, who denied her any interventions—including any dental work—which she badly needed. Since his death, Dusya had gone into therapy of her own accord, with urging from her husband. She was diagnosed with math dyslexia and later Asperger's. "I have learning difficulties, something like dyslexia but with numbers. I [also] have dyspraxia—I can't do anything with my fingers. I can't sew, I need help tying my shoe . . . I am name-blind, I have no knowledge of labels. But what I do have is a photographic memory. It's like I have a video camera in my head."

Dusya feels very strongly that there must be interventions and treatments that make sense for autistic people, whatever those approaches may be. She is particularly concerned that children get appropriate services, to teach them how to function as independently as possible. She pointed to the example of Stephen Shore, public speaker, educator, and autistic. Shore did not speak until late in childhood. Now as a public speaker and writer, he is an extremely accomplished man who has helped thousands on the spectrum—and their families—lead happier lives. Dedicated early intervention helped Shore begin to communicate. But this should be the rule, rather than the exception.

Because of Shore's example, Dusya believes passionately that colleges should offer accommodations, even options not to take certain tests, because many with Asperger's are very bright but no one believes it.

Dusya feels she was helped immensely by getting these diagnoses, and says it was a "huge relief":

When I was a child I had trouble with math, I thought that something was wrong with me . . . or that I wasn't trying hard enough. My teachers just kind of gave up, my father kept saying "No, no, no!" Whatever help I needed, he kept on saying "No." My father, even if I did something right, never told me good things. My father manipulated me . . . my mother manipulated me. Over thirty years, to hear that you are nothing, not good— it's hard to get rid of it.

Years later, her mother tried to apologize and explain why she could not be of more help to her daughter: "She told me, 'Dusya, I was crying, I was begging your father to get you help . . . he was God, he was the law.'" And so Dusya got no help; no therapy, dental work, or interventions for all of elementary, middle, and high school. "They just gave up. They couldn't help me. I didn't know what it was, I didn't know how to get help. Until I was seventeen, I couldn't even look people in the eye," she said. Processing, talking and thinking while looking people in the eye, is still hard for her. Yet as she moved into her late teens, Dusya wanted more for herself: she wanted college. However, certain family difficulties—again with her father—prevented that.

One afternoon, everything changed for Dusya. "Once, while my father was sleeping, I was watching a show where there was a little girl who was having trouble remembering things with math and I thought, *Oh my God she sounds so much like me!* Then my father had an accident, and I was the one who had to bring money to the house. I got a job as a nursing aide. But I wasn't able to work full time because my mother needed me as well."

Such wounds in childhood run deep. "I am angry, I am frustrated," she said. "Sometimes I got so angry with him . . . I wished I could kill him! After his death, I didn't want to think about him."

At some point into her twenties, however, Dusya realized how all the anger and terrible history was affecting her. I was a bit surprised at her degree of self-reflection. She found out about the Asperger's Association of New England, an advocacy and support group, and went there for game night. She met a young man there, and though they didn't even talk to each other that night, they soon fell in love. "He understands me," she says. "I need someone who can keep up with me intellectually. He can keep up with me." AANE had a social work intern who provided therapy. It was Dusya's new boyfriend who persuaded her to go. Dusya had previously resisted therapy, but not this time: she felt that the Asperger's Association people would provide a therapist who understood Asperger's syndrome.

Dusya's discovery of her own Asperger's and of the AANE was cathartic for her. Not only did she have a name, an explanation for her lifelong struggles and her feeling of difference: she found others who had gone through the same thing. It made me think how important it could be for everyone on the spectrum to learn about their diagnosis—how much it explains about their experiences! Of course, it is tough to know when the best time is to find out.

Another thing that struck me was the tug in her voice, the secret pleasure in her smile when she recounted these discoveries—how self-affirming and empowering her diagnoses were. And just then it hit me, what I'd been sensing for this entire interview: all this time, I'd been trying to be so delicate with her, so sensitive, because of her disability. Handle with care, this poor person has autism! But Dusya didn't need to be protected. *I* was the one who didn't get it. How many times do I have to learn the same thing? "You're proud of it, your Asperger's," I said.

"Yes." Then she said, "I don't want to boast, but it helps me see the world differently. Parents have a problem with saying their child is autistic. They don't like it if they think it's a disorder—I think that for them it's a disorder. I realize those parents, they cannot see . . . they want to *cure* autism." Dusya then softened a little: "I understand parents. They don't understand why their child is different. But even if we can't speak, we can go to college, we can do whatever. We can even be supermodels . . . I don't want to boast, but I think Aspies are out of the box." Dusya's pride in her diagnosis, and in her autistic peers, seemed almost like a tribal solidarity to me. To further illustrate how different neurological wiring can be advantageous, Dusya pointed to the iron gate at the subway stop, just outside our Starbucks. It was made of circular metal shapes and vertical bars. "If you would look at a gate, you would just see the gate. But I'm looking at those circles, and what it's made of."

Dusya then started to talk more about what mainstream society seems to think about autism. She doesn't like it. "I don't agree with Autism Awareness Month [which is in April]. *Everybody's* aware of autism! But they don't understand what it means. How it affects your brain. It's about understanding what it is the structure about it. How your brain works. Change it to Autism Understanding Month."

I wondered what Dusya would like to see in terms of autism understanding. What would she tell people, to make them understand autism better? Autism understanding is why I write. I use the example of Nat's life to show others a picture of autism. But for Dusya, it's about many pictures. It's about understanding the various manifestations of autism, along with all the possibilities and potential within autistics: "First of all, I think most normal people are ignorant about what autism is like. Even those who want to understand, most people when they think of autism, they think of Rain Man . . . the public puts us on the wrong side of autism. But autism has different phases. Think of Carly Fleischmann." Carly is a young Canadian woman who was non-verbal until she finally figured out how to express herself on a laptop. "Typing on a laptop, typing her feelings. She was highly intelligent, but nobody thought of this. Schools have to be educated," Dusya said. "They're ignorant. I really want our generation to have these possibilities. My dream is that in the future, children get *all* the accommodations wherever they want, for everything they are trying to study."

Married, autistic, and happy

"I seem like I don't have a disability," Bonnie told me. "I can drive, and perform most tasks with ease. I have a job and I'm married." Bonnie is a woman in her early thirties who lives in Oklahoma. She has had a particularly tough struggle for independence and to find happiness. She is diagnosed on the Asperger's end of the spectrum, and also with ADHD and clinical depression. She talked to me on the phone, asking me to change her name to protect her privacy.

"Is there something out there for an adult on the higher-functioning end? I don't require constant care, or any care, for that matter. I can take care of myself although I do struggle with organization. I mainly need someone to advocate for me in the job market and to help me stay organized," Bonnie said. Finding a job, staying organized on the job, all while dealing with the challenges of disability—these are the weak links for the most vulnerable in our society seeking work and independence.

Bonnie has also had a great degree of difficulty navigating boundaries with her mother, especially around money issues.

When I say 'money problems' and 'my mom,' I mean my mom asking my husband and me for money. She is extremely codependent and cannot function on her own. Terrance and I, on the other hand, are pretty good with our finances. When my mom calls me and wants me to do something for her, it's very difficult. She lives an hour and a half away. When she asks for money, that creates tension with my husband. I think about my mom; she's in a bad situation. I feel bad for her, and I can't help her. I get sad when I see women with their adult daughters, walking and talking and having a great time, because my mom can't walk. She gained a lot of weight; her knees are messed up beyond repair.

At the time of our interview, Bonnie had been married to Terrance for seven months in a house that Terrance bought a couple years before they'd met. Bonnie had not been looking to get married; she'd wanted a boyfriend. So she went onto the dating website OkCupid and found Terrance. "Prior to marriage, I lived in an apartment about a mile from my school that I found through a flyer at my school. I rented an apartment for two years."

Bonnie had two years of college, then later attended a vocational center where she studied information technology. The emphasis of the center was on networking.

"I worked in a restaurant and then saw an advertisement for an informational technology position. I got the job, but was let go five months later, over issues between me and my boss." Bonnie started a new job in IT recently, which is full time but with mandatory overtime—a required ten to fifteen hours a week overtime. Of course she receives overtime pay, but it is still a heavy workload.

"Right now, I don't have any support services," she said. It is not typical for a woman with her social, cognitive, and behavioral competence to get any help from public funding. That does not imply that Bonnie's life is easy. But she has worked very hard to find supports. "I just recently got on my husband's insurance. I have a large network of friends, people to lean on emotionally."

Bonnie has found that a lot of support groups for people with Asperger's, or autism for that matter, are not a good fit. However, if the support group also offers certain common bonds other than autism, Bonnie thrives.

I'm a part of numerous groups on Facebook; one is a group of people with Asperger's who have dogs and relationships, and some have people who are married. I'm able to get a lot of support from them. Most of my friends know about my diagnosis and what that is . . . Growing up, I had never been taught that who I was is OK. Parents, school, teachers, family members—I never got the message that I was OK. I had to change and be normal. Asperger's wasn't a diagnosis in 1983. In 1994, when I was ten, I got an 'unofficial' diagnosis of Asperger's. Because of insurance and funding, we couldn't get the paperwork done that we needed to get done so all the testing was put on hold.

While in school, the biggest problems Bonnie faced were bullying and staying organized. Being different was excruciating for her. "A few girls here and there would help me, by telling me things like 'don't do this, do this instead,' but mostly I had to handle the social codes on my own." She had to learn everything from what not to wear, to how to act in front of boys—an entire world of rules that are intricate, subtle, and change all the time.

Bonnie got her official diagnosis just months before she grad-uated high school. At that point, she received support and modi-fications that she'd badly needed. She had extended time on tests and was excused from pep rallies and other sensory-overload expe-riences. She also had permission to leave class and seek a school counselor whenever she felt overwhelmed emotionally.

Then, once she started college at Northeastern State University, the Department of Disabled Student Services provided her with testing modifications. But Bonnie also needed someone help plan her schedule, check in with her, and to make sure she was going to class and getting around OK. "I didn't know I needed that then," she said. "I would have graduated if I'd had those supports."

In 2010, Bonnie began to think about moving out to her own place, to get a healthier distance from her mother. "I started to go back to school, and I was spending more time at school with my classmates, or spending time at church, staying at friends' houses. I love my mom, but she's not the healthiest of people. I met friends who encouraged me to move out. And in March of 2011, I got my own place." Bonnie paid the rent through a work/study position and a job at McDonald's as a drive-through attendant. "Even with Asperger's I can work that drive-through," she said, "I like working." Her current job as a network tech-nician is very well compensated, with a comfortable salary and benefits. "I recognize that I have been blessed," wrote Bonnie.

Bonnie's relationship with her husband is a blissful part of her life. "I am a newlywed, and I think about my husband a lot. I like cuddling with him. I think about food, video games—Mario Cart, where you select different vehicles and race on different courses, that's my favorite game right now. I like to work out on the elliptical machines and with Wii Fit. If I could play any sport, it probably would be rugby or football because I like to be aggres-sive." She said this laughing.

Also, Bonnie enjoys chess and singing soprano in the city choir. "I like going to church. I leave a big impression on people. I was in a program called PATHWAYS . . . they give you a special song that represents what you are and I got 'What a Difference You Make in My Life,' by Ronnie Milsap."

Bonnie has found that she likes being a leader. "I lead a Celebrate Recovery Christian-based twelve-step group. We are taught that the twelve steps can be applied to any habit we're trying to overcome, such as compulsive behaviors that cause problems. I've always wanted to be a leader deep down inside . . . very often that was not an option for me . . . it took me a while to mature and to be the kind of person people would see as a leader."

Faith plays a large positive role in Bonnie's life.

I feel a lot of peace, a lot of comfort, like there's something driving me, that's controlling everything . . . I don't get my way every time . . . but I feel like my husband and me . . . someone's taking care of us, we're going to be fine. I worry that I won't be able to keep a high paying job and my husband will divorce me for it . . . irrational, but money stresses him out. I worry about having to move back in with my mom. Marriage is, for me, a victory. I love being married to Terrance. I love him with all my heart. But people on the autism spectrum don't get married very often. I'm doing something that people with my neurology have problems with. I feel like I'm a pioneer. I feel good, but I feel a lot of pressure on myself.

Bouncing back after a mostly difficult life

Kate was my college roommate thirty-two years ago at the University of Pennsylvania. At fifty-two, she has a diagnosis of Asperger's. Back then, she had difficulty expressing herself, fitting in, even making sense. She had some odd inflections, an almost British accent. She did not always know who I was. She sat in her room most of the time with the door shut. The suite phone would ring and I'd hear her saying, "I'll get it, I'll get it." But she wouldn't. Cruelly I would say, "So get it!" and then laugh. I knew nothing about autism at the time, and I did not understand her—nor did I try very hard. Mostly I ignored her, or even made jokes about her.

Years later she contacted me through my blog. I could scarcely believe this was the same person I'd known. I knew that I'd have to get her to talk to me for this book, but also for my own edification. I needed to connect with her and find some way to own my youthful meanness. To atone. Having Nat has taught me a lot about cruelty.

Kate was not necessarily interested in the subject of forgiveness, however. "You can't un-kill someone who has been murdered," she said, giving me the chills. Nevertheless, I am so grateful that she granted me this interview, to help both people as clueless as I was and younger generations with autism, so that maybe they won't suffer the way she did.

Kate had changed so dramatically since our days in college. She was so reflective and wise about how things were for her then—so much for the stereotype of the autistic who cannot reflect on himself. I wondered how she had evolved to this point.

Kate talked for over an hour with very few moments for me to break in. Her speech ran fast and linear, each thought linked inextricably to the other. "Hard for me to say," Kate began.

I feel as if I was the same person inside but I did not have a channel whereby to express it. I was at home until I married my husband, Andy. My parents and his hooked us up, right after I self-diagnosed with Asperger's and had told my parents. They agreed I was right. They said, "You know Andy, he was at your bat mitzvah; his parents know us, we know him a lot better than you, and we think you have so much in common. You've never really been in a long term relationship."

Kate's parents helped her get out of the house and make a life for herself. "I'd had a job or two at that time, Dilbert-type office jobs, that I was good at but not exactly happy at," she said. After she left Penn she got an MLS and got a job in a high school in a drug- and gang-ridden Brooklyn slum. The place was raw with violence; a teacher was shot twenty feet from her.

Kate talked about how she always felt a kind of sub rosa hostility toward her at the school that she could not explain. She referred to that particular work experience as "Kafka-esque," where it felt at times that her colleagues were lying to her about things—tricking her. She'd be left off rosters, excluded from invitations to meetings and events, and then scolded for not knowing about them. Eventually this came to a head when her supervisors decided suddenly to fire her. "They said I *somehow* wasn't working out, but they couldn't put their finger on it." Even though she had tried to follow all procedures, rules, and appropriate behaviors of a staff person, they brought up issues about her performance that to Kate were grossly unfair. "People said, 'Kate is not evil or incompetent. None of this looks like Kate's fault, but I just have a *feeling* that she is not doing things the right way.'" School personnel said this, even though there was documentation that Kate had taught several students how to read, getting them from "little or no alphabet knowledge" to "comprehending third-grade material." Kate had also taught eighteen students to write more effectively in terms of both content and handwriting through a lunchtime club she ran called the "Handwriting and Calligraphy Club."

Kate's contract was not renewed, and she left that job feeling utterly betrayed by her colleagues and not understanding what or why that had happened. I suspect that this is the kind of experience that dogs many people on the autism spectrum in the working world.

But still, I could not figure out how Kate had gone from being my eighteen-year-old roommate shut into her bedroom, friendless, bizarre, and alone, to this self-possessed, married public speaker and advocate. I felt I needed to harness Kate's fiery energy and get her to reflect on her progress. I wanted to forge all this information into direct help for younger autism families facing adulthood. But sometimes a good story is the most effective lesson, and that was what Kate was giving me.

"I left Penn as a junior and I was at home again. Since I was someone who was doing my best to do everything I was told, if you told me, 'You're too stupid to do something,' I would not rebel. I was trying to be a grownup. I was hitting bottom as far as life tasks."

But then a remarkable opportunity opened up for her, from her deep interest in handwriting, of all things. "I had the chance to read the history of handwriting during grad school," she said. "Some accounts were recent enough that the authors were still alive, so I could write to them." She eventually became well known for her knowledge of handwriting and as a handwriting teacher.

"There wasn't any grand epiphany," she said, considering my question about her incredible development into adulthood. "It was simply that I had an endeavor on my own: the handwriting. I'd grown up with people screaming at me, 'You write like an epileptic. You write like your aunt Eileen who is in a wheelchair.' I was my first student. My father became my second student, as his handwriting had been an issue forever. Once he saw this was not some crazy thing and I was not just a crazy person, once they saw that this was actually interesting and effective, it was harder for them to see me as a lazy, stupid monstrosity. It was my father who made the suggestion that I offer my services to doctors. 1996—the year they introduced Viagra and people were writing three hundred scrips a day."

I'd like to note here that Kate asked me to try to come up with a different description of parents like me, saying that she found the term autism parents to be "creepy." I stand by my word choice, however, because I have not had pushback from the majority of those I've interviewed.

Eventually Kate came up with some good advice for autism parents and caregivers:

The biggest is to make sure that you are not defining success so narrowly that it is not possible for success to exist. The problem was when I'd look for jobs in the paper, and find things I was qualified to apply for, and my parents would say, '" don't want you in a lousy job, I want you in a good job." I felt like I was trying to cross the Grand Canyon on a bridge, a wire one molecule wide, and that molecule was being shaved down from the left and then from the right. I was not allowed to stand still or go backward, I could only go forward.

As autism researchers Lynn Kerns Koegel and Peter Gerhardt advise, Kate emphasized the importance of looking for vocational interests in the autistic penchant for obsession. "You need to look at what interests and abilities the person has, as opposed to the interests and abilities you want him to have. If he plays Dungeons and Dragons, maybe you have to help find him a job working with people to make an app for the iPad. You may be able to take some of them and see if the local cub scout troop can learn games that tie into merit badges. Even if it's raking leaves or flipping burgers. There are no lousy jobs, there are only lousy people who tell you this job is no good."

Along with striving to be supportive and encouraging of your autistic loved one's interests, Kate felt parents and caregivers must be careful about what it is they expect. She cautioned against expectations that set one up for failure. "My parents wanted me to be Jewish, to have a Jewish education. But they never really defined that. There were some things that were important to them, some things that were not, so when I kept kosher and they would say, 'We wanted you to be Jewish but not *too* Jewish.' I would say, 'Well, tell me what percentage Jewish you want me to be?'"

I pressed Kate to give me specifics about what parents should *not* do. She said, "Never put the kid in a situation where they might feel you are gaslighting them," she said, referring to the many times in her own life when she would feel "gaslighted"—a person would do or say something hurtful, and then compound this by telling her, "Do not see this as harm or punishment, or pain."

Another point Kate made was about being up-front in terms of sexuality and basic human needs. "You have to be prepared: the kid is going to grow up and is going to be physically mature and have sex. You have to talk about this." Kate knew a mother who had a sixteen-year-old daughter with Down syndrome, who was really creeped out by her daughter's sexual development. Apparently the mother said, "She's getting her period, she's got breasts! I thought that because her development was slowed, her development would be slowed! Now she talks about boys, I had to take her bra-shopping! I did not think I'd have to deal with this." Kate was incredulous and outraged by this mother's ignorance, probably because it reminded her of her own mother's attitude toward her sexuality. Kate said, "I was not on good enough terms with my mom that I could talk about sex and contraceptives, even though I'd been going to doctors on my own. I didn't really know what the social protocol was for asking for a referral to go to a gynecologist."

Toward the end of our conversation, Kate said, "No one should be punished for seeing life through their own prism. I would say, 'Parents of autistic anyone, you need to figure this out: what does it take to rear your child as a human being, instead of a lab rat, a performing dog, or some kind of indoor cat?' Everyone is diminished by inhumane treatment."

Resources to simplify life on the autism spectrum:

- *The Unwritten Rules of Social Relationships: Decoding Social Mysteries Through the Unique Perspectives of Autism,* Dr. Temple Grandin and Sean Barron, both of whom are well-known and beloved autistic authors (Future Horizons, 2005).

- *A 5 Is Against the Law! Social Boundaries: Straight Up! An Honest Guide for Teens and Young Adults,* Karri Dunn Buron (Autism Asperger Publishing Company, 2007).
- *The Integrated Self-Advocacy ISA™ Curriculum: A Program for Emerging Self-Advocates with Autism Spectrum and Other Conditions,* Valerie Paradiz (Autism Asperger Publishing Company, 2009).
- *The Hidden Curriculum of Getting and Keeping a Job: Navigating the Social Landscape of Employment: A Guide for Individuals With Autism Spectrum and Other Social-Cognitive Challenges,* Brenda Smith Myles, Judy Endow, and Malcolm Mayfield (Autism Asperger Publishing Company, 2012).
- *Intimate Relationships and Sexual Health: A Curriculum for Teaching Adolescents/Adults with High-Functioning Autism Spectrum Disorders and Other Social Challenges,* Catherine Davies and Melissa Dubie, MS (Autism Asperger Publishing Company, 2011).
- *Learning the Hidden Curriculum,* Judy Endow (Autism Asperger Publishing Company, 2012).
- *A Freshman Survival Guide for College Students with Autism Spectrum Disorders,* Haley Moss (Jessica Kingsley, 2014).
- *Sexuality and Safety with Tom and Ellie* book series, Kate E. Reynolds, Jonathon Powell (Jessica Kingsley, 2014).

CHAPTER SEVEN

AUTISTIC ADULTS WITH COMMUNICATION OR APPARENT COGNITIVE CHALLENGES

"Live in 'parment."

> —Nat's answer, when given the choice between moving to an apartment or staying in a group home

WHAT IS THE KEY TO helping our guys have happy, dignified lives? If I were to come up with one fairly universal answer, I would say, "The ability to communicate." Communication seems to be the dividing line in terms of outward functioning ability. If you can talk, converse, ask questions, you can likely be more included in society, in school, and in jobs. But it's not actually that simple. If your speaking is compromised by social skill challenges, disruptive behavior, or emotional struggle, then you may face terrible obstacles out in the world.

What is it like for the communication-impaired or even cognitively delayed autistic adult? How do they express themselves, their wants, needs, and dreams? In my case, I observe Nat intently and I try to prompt him to let me know what is going on inside him when he needs to. I have only moderate success, though. Whether this is because he cannot connect with his own feelings and then express them, or because perhaps he doesn't want to tell me, I do not get clarity from Nat very often.

And how is it for others with family members like Nat? I turned to families with loved ones whose diagnosis could be thought of as "severe" in one way or another. This was a particularly challenging chapter to write because of the very nature of the severity of their diagnosis—how do you talk to someone who cannot communicate? Or whose perspective or experiences are greatly limited by their autism? As I found in the previous chapter, each family has its own unique story, but it is possible to pick out connecting points for ourselves and learn from each other.

Nat's communication evolution/revolution

I believe that improving communication ability can be a step toward improving a difficult or isolated life. How could it not be? Once you can tell others what is going on, or ask questions, you can learn and you can grow. You can become more comfortable with the world around you if you understand it. This was the case with Nat. I discovered that Nat was interested in typing if it was in a context, a structure. Like everything else in his life, he needed to see and understand the boundaries, the outlines, and the conventions of any given activity. Many fellow autism moms began urging me to get Nat an iPad, saying he could communicate through it. I was reluctant because I thought that Nat just could not link the concept of computer activity with speaking. He had only rarely played video games, and he showed little interest in using the computer to learn. He did type the occasional email with heavy support from his teachers, but he did not seem to enjoy it. But things changed during 2012, and I wrote about it for the *Washington Post:*

> *One recent afternoon we weren't doing much; I was online, checking email and Facebook. For no particular reason, I called Nat over to look at my Facebook page. He must have been bored, for he came right away. He seemed fascinated with the little thumbnail images of all the people I know—many of whom he knows as well. An idea began to bloom.*
>
> *"Hey, Nat," I said, "you want to type on my Facebook page here?" To my surprise, he answered yes. I had no idea what to expect and sat back while Nat's finger hovered over the keyboard, his thoughts slowly coalescing into words. He'd finally shout a word out and I'd say, "Okay, type that!" Then he'd sound it out, using the invented spelling of kindergartners—but this was anything but babyish.*
>
> *Seeing Nat's words on the screen felt miraculous. One of the first things he typed was—not surprisingly—"look at pikerts" (look at pictures). I posted a note on my Facebook wall that Nat was typing. Moments later, responses began pouring in. It seemed like all my Facebook friends wanted to talk to Nat. I asked Nat if he wanted to say something back. He typed some responses: "hi" and "how you." I wanted to shout, jump, and kiss him all at once but I stopped myself. I had waited many years for communication like this, but my son was a twenty-two-year-old man at the time. I encouraged him, but quietly, the way he needs it to be.*
>
> *Nat and I soon created his own Facebook account—with him doing most of the typing. In sending out friend requests, I invited his two brothers, a tricky venture because they did not want to friend me or their father. But Max accepted Nat right away, without a word. And he has been "liking" posts on Nat's page.*
>
> *Nat's is just one Facebook page out of nearly a billion. But in our family, glaciers are melting and mountains moving. My younger son asked me the other day why I had put Nat on*

Facebook. I thought for a moment, then told him the truth: "I don't know. It just seems like he's ready to join the rest of the world."

"Okay, I'll friend him," he said. Four little words, but sometimes that's all you need.

For Nat, Facebook is the best way to talk through typing. He can look at his friends and choose to post a message to any of them, and if they are online at the moment, they will respond. Facebook has provided Nat with his first manageable conversational medium.

Because Nat was able to tell us occasional things about himself—provided we asked first, and structured the questions in ways he could answer—we learned that he did want to live in an apartment, as I discussed previously.

Once we knew this was what he wanted, and we had John's commitment to be his caregiver, we started looking for apartments in the urban, more affordable neighborhoods in Boston—what I fondly call the "student slums." They are not actual slums; they are more like ghettos of students and shabby apartments that so many of us get for our first homes after dorm life.

I found a place that John and Nat could afford within the DDS's guidelines. It was a small two bedroom, newly renovated. I got busy with buying Nat cute, cheap furniture at Home Goods. We moved him in on June 1, 2014.

A few words go a long way

When Evan said "Roll Tide" to me, I at first wasn't sure what I had heard.

His mother Marikay explained, "That would be 'Roll Tide.' That's Alabama, by the way: the Crimson Tide cheer is 'Roll Tide.' Sometimes we really do say Roll Tide around here rather than hello. That's our favorite thing to do this time of year."

Evan is twenty-eight years old, diagnosed on the autism spectrum. He lives with his family: mother, stepfather, sister, and her three small children. During our conversation, Marikay sat with Evan, sometimes interpreting his mostly one-word verbal answers, but usually I could understand him, after I'd gotten used to his Southern accent. He is a low-pitched and infrequent speaker, often completely quiet. He reminded me of Nat because of his dependence on others to help him communicate at all, and yet unlike Nat, he can initiate conversations and react to others' comments. When you read this, imagine a soft voice and a long, deep Southern drawl.

Evan first told me, after some prompting and waiting, that he has been working since he left school, around seven years ago. He also worked while he was in school—in the kitchen at a Marriott hotel, loading and unloading the dishwasher.

Evan currently packs medical kits part-time for his job, but this is not done in a sheltered workshop, nor through any agency. Marikay, his mom, told me that his job is in a local company, where the employer is someone who knows Evan and his family. There is no one else involved. The company owner was familiar enough with Even and his skill in concentrating that he simply hired him, with no Department of Developmental Services help—he would not qualify for that level of support, or funding, and certainly not a job coach (although he'd had one when he first entered adulthood). He is still considered under the umbrella of one state vocational program that offers job coaching as needed. Someone from that service provider calls every other month to check on his job status and ask if he needs help.

Recently, the company where Evan works was sold to another company. "We have been reassured that the three special needs young adults (which include Evan) will continue to be part of what has always been a family-type business," said Marikay.

Evan has a real community around him, actual neighbors and friends who support him. Evan told me that during his day he eats a snack at work. He also has two friends at work, Pete and

Donald. I did not know what sort of friendships Evan might be capable of or interested in, so I asked him what Pete and Donald do at their jobs. There was a pause, and Marikay had to answer for Evan. She said that Pete is a supervisor in the workplace, and Donald is the helper. The young workers only do four-hour shifts at a time, because it's tiring and kind of tedious. So the other young adults do not get the opportunity to form a natural social network with Evan because they come in Tuesdays and Thursdays when Evan is not there. Because of their differing hours, he does not see them much.

To compensate for Evan's lack of social life during the work-week, Marikay found him things to do with others during the weekend. "Can you tell her about the party on the mountain?" Marikay asked him.

"I get my Saturday nights out," Evan answered slowly, though readily and clearly.

Marikay then elaborated for him, "It's one Saturday a month with the kids he's known forever that he plays ball with. They go to a gym. Evan has also been active with his Miracle League baseball team since he was eleven. He has now moved up to the adult league. He enjoys both the spring and fall baseball seasons."

On the other Saturdays, Evan visited his dad.

"I see my dad. I go out to his house," Evan replied. Evan—through Marikay's encouragement, intervention, and interpretation—also told me that he does not go to the movies because the sound is too loud. Instead, he and his dad watch baseball. They like to watch the Braves and, of course, the Crimson Tide football games.

Evan and Marikay live with Evan's sister and her three children, two of whom, though they are very little, are twins who have been diagnosed with autism, too. Evan told me their names—Marissa and Weston and Vivi—and that he likes to be around them. "The kids climb all over their Uncle Evan, and he sits calmly and happily while they do," said Marikay. "The youngest, three-year-old Vivi, has recently been diagnosed with a newly discovered genetic disorder involving developmental delays."

At one point Evan told me that the thing that makes him happiest is to go on the swing in his yard. Marikay remarked that she'd kept him really busy that morning. He'd taken the garbage down to the garbage can, he'd put the can onto the street, and he'd emptied the dishwasher. "He's very willing to do things I ask him to do. I'm grateful for that," she said.

Even though Marikay does a lot of advocating with her daughter for the autistic twins, she is currently not pursuing additional help for Evan. She feels that his life is going smoothly now in his adulthood, while she is desperately worried about her daughter, whose three children all have recently diagnosed special needs. "Evan is actually the easiest person to deal with in the house," she said with a smile in her voice.

Verbal, smart, but still struggling

I've known Pete and his family for twenty-one years. Pete's mom was in my first support group. She told me the story of "green," to show me just how Pete thought as a four-year-old. Lisa was walking with Pete down a school corridor, full of people and sounds, surrounded by long walls full of notices, artwork, and posters. As they moved down the hall, Pete suddenly said, "Green." *Green?* Lisa thought. There was nothing green there. There were many colors on those walls. But Pete said, again, "Green." And he walked up to a tiny, tiny dot of green in the middle of all that chaotic color and paper. Green.

Pete is now in his twenties, and he was living in a group home at the time of this interview, after a short, disastrous stint in a different group home. Lisa hated the first group home for him because there was no one there—staff or resident—who could give Pete what he really needed, which competent oversight. Pete himself knew about the need to find just the right group home, and the dangers others face in poorly run residences: "I have heard of group homes not very often reported on in newspapers, or foster care systems where they abuse people," he said. Lisa felt that in the first group home, the problem was that Pete had no peers there in any sense; the others were in their forties.

Pete needs guidance for the gray areas of life. Lisa said, "One time I came home from work to a house full of smoke. Peter was in the house, but did not notice all the smoke and when I told him he had left the burner on he said, 'Really?'" Pete believes these things happened because of his health condition which left him foggy-minded and weak. Pete had been debilitated by certain dietary issues of which none of them had been aware. "He'd lost thirty pounds, becoming so thin at one point he could not walk," Lisa told me, "and also he began developing his first grand mal seizures."

This was a horrible low point in the family's life. The situation was very difficult for Lisa, who does not know how to help him manage his struggle with periodic mental health issues that hinder his ability to understand what he can and cannot do in life. At times, Lisa and her husband Dan have been truly at a loss for what would be best for Pete in terms of family stress levels and safety. Although Pete can express himself and function well in many areas, he can get into trouble because people don't realize his deficits in social comprehension. He can get into situations where he is too trusting of strangers, too gullible, and may not be safe out in the community for too long. Lisa and Pete have been in search of a staff person who is kind of like a friend, who can guide him while not making him feel like he was being babysat. Like Nat, he also needs schedules, and many prompts and cues for daily living activities like showering, eating and drinking properly, and self-care on other levels.

Challenges aside, Pete did go to a year of community college, and would love to do more; yet when Lisa tried to get him to try any new classes, he declined. But he still insists that he will go to law school, or become a realtor, or even a scientist—he has dreams like all of us, but it is far harder for him to manage what he envisions with what his true abilities and issues are. Lisa despairs that he will not be able to realistically attain these goals, and she doesn't know how to talk to him about more realistic ones.

I have heard Lisa's point of view for years, but I had never talked directly to Pete. He is very intense, and I had been a little intimidated by the idea of interviewing him. I did not know if he would get stuck on a subject that I knew nothing about, if the conversation would drag on and on, or if he would get upset with me. I had no idea if I could connect with him or get him to open up. But I also worried that if he did open up, it might make him sad about his life. Nevertheless, I made contact with him through Facebook and arranged to interview him.

He described himself as follows: "I'm different from normal people, but I'm not that much different. Like I can make a better meal than my staff."

Pete feels that he can help his housemates, too, perhaps even more effectively than the staff there. He tries to advise some of the others in his group home who may need help understanding things around them, and he is aware of how they may feel about getting help from him: "It can be embarrassing for one of my other housemates, like when I give him smart advice because his planning doesn't make sense. I try to help, but he is embarrassed because he is twenty-eight and I'm twenty-five. It's backwards because I know more things but he is older, so the world is Opposite Day."

Pete is also (deservedly) proud of other skills he has, with assembling things and cooking. "I put together all my furniture from Ikea in my first group home—desk, dresser, chair, nightstand, and lamp—with almost no staff help. Just following all the directions. I have a tool box in my house, so I fixed my roommate's pot with a screwdriver and I fixed the toilet pipe with a wrench." He also told me he shops for himself. And he gets places independently, and cooks delicious-sounding meals for himself: "I can cook on my own, with no help. I can make chicken broccoli ziti, Asian stir fry, grilled tuna melt, eggs, omelets, chicken cacciatore, fish, scallops, and Mediterranean chicken. I can cook by using liquor, like red wine, vodka, and rum, I can make beer-battered wings. I can make Trinidad recipes that require four-hour cooking. I can bake, too."

I was enchanted, mesmerized, and at times moved to tears by Pete talking and writing to me about his life. No matter how much I think I know autism and people, both are always surprising me.

Pete spoke in a monotone, without many breaks or pauses. He was able, however, to stop when I cut in and asked him questions. He told me that his life's dream was to pass the GED and then maybe go to a trade school. "I don't have my GED because I put my dream to the hold because I wanted my health to get better so I could focus. Now I am practicing with a GED book." He did not graduate with a diploma because Massachusetts, like most states, ties graduation to passing a standardized test. The federal Elementary and Secondary Education Act, known as No Child Left Behind, created an obstacle to graduating because school systems were under pressure to be sure all students would be able to read and do math at a particular level—whether they had a disability or English was their second language. Most states choose to measure literacy and numeracy by one standardized test, and so students with any sort of test-taking trouble or comprehensive disabilities stood to be, well, left behind by being denied diplomas.

Pete said, "I did not get the best education in school because it was too much like kindergarten. All they did was play wheel of fortune and color on paper instead of learning academics and money skills. So I graduated and learned almost nothing, so I don't have a GED or diploma. So I want to go back to school for my GED."

Lisa takes seriously his desire to get his GED, yet she is not sure how best to help Pete. Indeed, it may be even harder for her to help him because he has so many opinions about himself and what he wants—whether they are realistic ideas or not. In some ways, it is easier for me to deal with Nat because his challenges are not about mental health. The combination of an autism spectrum disorder and mental health are becoming more frequently recognized, but society is a long way from knowing how to help those with problems like Pete's.

Pete told me that he wanted to live on his own in an apartment in one of the more suburban neighborhoods nearby. He was leery of living in "projects," which I suppose was a reference to Section 8 housing, or perhaps general "institutional" places like group homes. As he put it, "I don't want to be around where there's a lot of crime rates." He talked about how he would someday maybe buy his own house.

But there could be potential disastrous pitfalls if Pete were to live on his own. He may not fully understand how his disability, and his inconsistent grasp of certain social interactions, could get in the way or get him in trouble. Although he does have some idea of what he might confront: "What if the landlord is a big jerk . . . should I be honest with a boss if he asks me to be honest, or should I lie . . . I like being honest with people," he said, giving me an Impressionist-like picture of his multicolored pervasive anxiety. But I could see how this type of quandary and forthrightness would hinder him in this complicated world.

Pete wears his feelings heavily on his thin frame, and he experiences his ill-fitted situations acutely. He does not want unproductive days. But things are starting to change. "My DDS worker is really good and understands my case, so he is trying to find a different program," Pete said. "I only like my day program a little, but it's better than the programs I went to before. Now there are not only nonverbal people there."

He told me that if he could go to school again, eventually he'd be able to find his own job: "Well, I know that I'm too old to go back to high school, but I know there are programs." He told me he'd taken classes at a community college but it wasn't enough because he still needed to learn more community skills. Pete had felt comfortable there, though; there were some special classes for people with disabilities, yet were not segregated:

they would mix it up a little with people without disabilities. So why couldn't he go back there? Again I could feel his frustration. "Instead of sitting in a warehouse, I would like to do something like learn what I should do in an independent situation." His phrasing and cadences, though unusual, conveyed perfectly how he felt about his life: how much of it was beyond his control, and this stung him.

I wanted to hug Pete, to be the big mommy and fix everything. But he has a terrific mom already. It's just that his dreams are so like what I have for Nat, and what Nat now has. But Pete can express this where Nat cannot. And yet, what good does that do him, if his other challenges limit him—including his ability to understand his own limitations. (Pete maintains that he does understand his challenges; Lisa, on the other hand worries that he does not.)

The flawed adult services system frustrates Lisa to no end. She feels that Pete could do much better if people would only offer him options that fit his true abilities. "I think Pete could work as a helper or an apprentice to a contractor or landscaper. He is such a good worker. Every boss he has ever had has told me how hard-working Pete is. He might not be able to work completely independently, but he could work alongside someone."

Currently, Pete has a job working in a bowling alley, but he wants more than this for himself. "No specifics, but some ideas are: house designing, landscaping, computer technology, real estate, or private investigator."

Pete has been on a special diet, and he has gotten stronger since those dark days of malnourishment in his first group home. The diet is complicated and demanding, but he has been able to follow it nevertheless, and told me more about the body chemistry involved than I could understand. But the restrictions chafe at him. He said that if he wasn't on that diet, he probably would like to go out to eat at the Cheesecake Factory, Chili's, or maybe a pizza place, "where they have a twelve-inch slice, or a fifteen-inch slice. I still have good taste in food; I'm not a picky eater at all and I also used to take the bus to the place," he said, in his typical stream-of-consciousness style. Because of his GI issues, however, he usually saw friends after dinner, which he also did not like. "But," he said, "I don't want to get the shakes and pass out."

I felt sad about the lack of choice Pete seemed to have in his life. I wondered about how this felt to him. I have had to be careful not to project my feelings on others I've interviewed, especially people with autism who have a very different perception of things. My empathy might be misplaced, unwelcome, or even patronizing.

Still thinking about food, Pete told me that at the moment his mother was baking pumpkin bread for him. "I am pretty grateful that she's baking it," he said. "I'm thankful anyway, even though it doesn't taste like real bread. I think of it in a way like having a prosthetic arm. The gluten is the real body part." I think anyone on a gluten-free diet would probably agree: it's just not as much fun using substitutes in one's life. But Pete did not come off as self-pitying; he just told it like it was. "At least I don't have diabetes. I do have to worry about gluten, but my situation could have been worse. At least I can have fruit."

Pete has a great attitude, a lot of insight, and a good sense of humor to carry him through many difficulties. Still, I am afraid that he is one of those people who will fall through the cracks. He knows too much about the world and yet not nearly enough. Pete is exactly the kind of autistic person that our system has to learn to care about, and to develop supports suited for his special needs: autism and mental health challenges. One size does not fit all—not for school exit exams, day programs, diets, and certainly not for disabilities like autism.

When he can't speak for himself

In writing this book, one of my biggest concerns was to represent the autism spectrum at its fullest. There are many books written for people with Asperger's and "high-functioning" autism, but not many about guys like Nat, who cannot be left alone, who have difficulty communicating, and who may have challenging behaviors. I wanted to be able to convey what life is or could be like for even these "low-functioning" folks, and for most of this book, I interviewed loved ones and caregivers to get that information. But this chapter is supposed to be about autistics themselves—how they see their lives, what they have experienced, and what they hope for. I wanted to capture their voices.

But how do you capture the voice of someone who is nonverbal or, for the most part, non-communicative? I've spent all of Nat's life trying to get inside his head and understand what life is like for him. It did not seem practical for me to do this with strangers, especially those who have difficulty understanding the world around them.

So I did what I thought was the next best thing. I talked to one of my oldest friends who has an adult son with autism like Nat, but with even more challenges (I have changed their names and state to protect the privacy of the family and especially William, who cannot speak for himself). I have known Karen's son William all his life. He has always reminded me of Nat. William has profound difficulty expressing himself. Off and on, he has had trouble controlling aggressive behavior. He turned twenty-one recently, and has just finished with school. To an outside observer, William might appear to be very much in his own world. He's tall with bright floating curls, and he has his mother's sharp eyes. The last time he visited us, he had trouble feeling calm and he jumped up and down in our living room. He may have scared my youngest son, Ben, a bit. He certainly unsettled me, because I'd been there before, with Nat having the same kind of stormy, unpredictable mood. Later on, though, right after dinner, he and Nat shared a laugh over their ice cream. That sweet moment tells me a lot. There is no doubt about it: there is so much going on in our guys' minds.

Karen told me a bit about William because, of course, he cannot tell me himself. To me, William represents that part of the autism spectrum that is seldom taken into account: those with many autistic symptoms, who cannot communicate much, and who have cognitive, sensory, and behavioral challenges.

Yet right away, Karen wanted to qualify that assessment of her son: "William is very social, albeit mostly silently. You can find him at a party or with a big group of people, hanging around on the edge. He wants to be near them. This comes from how long he has lived happily in a big community."

William may be unreadable to those who don't know him, but he is not as big a mystery to Karen, his family, and his school community. He loves listening to music and going for bike rides—on a tandem bike, because he's not a reliable driver. He loves going for car rides, swimming, and taking hikes.

In Pennsylvania, when you turn twenty-one you stop being the school district's responsibility. At the time of this interview, William was about to enter adult services, and Karen's main task has been to find him a day program and a residential setting that will meet his social and vocational needs—a process that for Karen has been extremely disappointing. She's found adult services disorganized and difficult to understand. "Everyone gives you a separate piece of info," she said. "But at least we have a service coordinator who helps us piece the bits together somewhat." This helpful coordinator has service providers that she likes, and she steers Karen toward them. From there, Karen asks around and others tell her about more residential and day places to check out.

"We are in an inchoate phase," Karen told me. "Constantly going around looking at day programs, community living scenarios."

Ideally, William's adult setting would be similar to the program he has been in since he was a teen, which is a farm community. Living on a farm, there's a very intense rhythm to the entire year, in a community with a lot of people—some are helpers, and some need more help. In William's teen setting, there had been no strong differentiation between clients and providers. There they are equals. That's what he's used to. The neurotypical people in his community have a vocation for communal living and for living with people with special needs. They enjoy it, and want to do it. They make jokes about them like they're good friends, and have a real life. "That's hard to replicate," said Karen. "Sadly we cannot provide that for William in our own home. It does take a lot of helpers." Unfortunately, the farm community nearest to them does not accept government funding; it is private pay only, which is exorbitantly expensive. Karen finds this to be incredibly unfair and bad practice. "From the practical point of view, these kinds of communities cost far less than typical group homes," Karen believes, "particularly when you consider that the day program is a natural part of the setup. But because the farm organization needs to do it this way—their own way—and because they don't want the regulations that accompany public funding, they must remain privately funded." Because none of these communities accept people who need the level of care William does, going into debt in order to provide a healthy living situation for their son is a moot point. Although they applied to the local adult farm community, despite the economic challenge it would pose, William was rejected for not being independent enough.

Determining what William wants in life is a big challenge for Karen, of course. She wants him to be able to take part in his own life decisions, "But I'm not sure he realizes very much about it at all. We have taken him to several interviews, and he always seems very much like, 'Okay, what am I doing here, can I get something to eat?' Not sure how much he really understands. Once we have something set, we'd do social stories and multiple visits to acclimate him"—similar to what my friend Cheryl and her team did for Nicky's doctor's visits.

Strong rhythm and structure to the day is key for William. Karen said, "He can do a lot of stuff on his own once the rhythm is established; what to do, where to bring things. We're looking for a situation that has a set rhythm to the day. At his farmstead school, they believe in work. Everyone needs to do work and do real work." And William can do a lot: he can make his bed, put clothes in the hamper, sort clothes into colors, darks, and whites, and he can put some of his laundry away. He works at home in other ways as well, helping a little bit with cooking, setting the table, and moving tables and chairs around. "He also did work outside on the farm, pushing a wheelbarrow, hefting rocks, moving branches. He helps grow garlic, mulches and waters (in the greenhouse). He even herds the cows, walking with them—and they follow him, probably because he's so big," Karen said, laughing.

Karen has been surprised by the different attitudes she has come across in some of the adult day programs she has visited. "Some seem great! But in some I get the feeling that they're simply babysitting or taking care of these people, with little engagement or expectation."

Karen and I talked a bit about the line between self-determination, eliciting William's own wants and needs, and letting him make unhealthy choices. There needs to be a balance, she has learned, because he may gorge himself on too much sugar and fat or just sit around if she were to take self-determination to the extreme. He and Nat do need supervision and guidance. We need to be their guardians in every sense of the word, because Nat and William's judgment skills and cognitive abilities are limited. She said, "William might be very happy to sit around, but I don't think that's good for him. If he were able to talk, he'd maybe say, 'I want to sit around listening to music while you cook for me, then take a long car ride and get-soft serve ice cream.'" This characterization might make some self-advocates angry, but Karen is being honest about William's perceived abilities and desires. It is her duty to help and protect him, her precious child. "He does not appear to have any understanding of future consequences. He'd sit there and eat twenty desserts. You could ask, 'William, do you like doing this job,' and he'd say 'Yes,' or 'No,' and it may not be true. In any given situation or interaction, we don't know how much he understands. So his true likes and dislikes are hard to know."

In the end, you have to know your guy well. I have to observe Nat and spend a lot of time with him to keep current with his skills and preferences. Karen does the same.

At one group home, we felt like we wanted William to do chores, and they said, 'Yes, no problem, if it was in his ISP. [Individualized Support Plan].' The day programs really vary a lot. [We need] one where they have a strong rhythm to their days, other than holidays. This on this day, that on that day. This kind of schedule helps William understand his environment and feel happier, calmer, more productive, and have the most satisfying interactions with others.

The programs Karen and her husband Rob ended up feeling best about were a mix of actual work, maybe even getting paid, and other structured activities. "If the clients seemed excited and happy, then we felt happy." At some places, people were coming up to her, excited to tell a visitor about their piece work jobs of assembling small gadgets: "Hey, I did two hundred of these yesterday!" Still, to have people initiating conversation like that implies a different cluster of skills, and that it might not be a good fit for William.

I thought about all of the work and daily living skills William had clearly learned at the farm school. What would happen to all of those skills in a program where he sits around staring at a big screen TV and eating Cheetos, singing with staff? The low expectations and scant developmental opportunities are what I personally hate about most day habilitation programs.

Karen acknowledged that in these programs, there's a lot of minimally satisfying conditions you do have to accept, like time spent celebrating sports events your kid may have no interest in. "Clearly, you have to be open-minded," she said, "and accept that every program has its own unique culture, and that's not a bad thing." Her hope is to find a program with flexible, intelligent, sensitive staff and managers and a consistent structure. "I am trying to retrofit things," she said, meaning she will work with them to make William's program more tailored to him, and she will work on the ISP to that end as well.

But it's all up in the air, and she has no idea what the future will really look like. Like most parents in the "falling off the cliff" year, she is living with total uncertainty about what her son's post-graduation life will look like.

Yet, being Karen, a mom who really knows her guy inside and out, she admitted that William probably would not mind just sitting around some. I know the same is true for Nat; on his weekends home with us, he spends a lot of time going from couch to couch. "But somehow," she said, "in these places that are not our home, that thought seems very much more sad." And then she said, with her characteristic wry humor—perhaps the most important ingredient of all in successful autism parenting—"So I will also look for a place that has nice couches."

CHAPTER EIGHT

AM I MY BROTHER'S KEEPER?

I am the youngest brother of someone with "severe" autism. At an early age I was exposed to his violent outbursts and in many instances was hurt in the process. I was diagnosed with a form of PTSD at a shockingly early age. I grew up with hatred. Disgust for him for the things I had to endure. I was confused. It was a dark time for all of us.

I grew to love Nat unconditionally as a brother, and in turn have learned that he is one of the sweetest people you could ever meet, despite occasional, sometimes violent outbursts and years of nonverbality."

—Ben, Nat's youngest brother

THE AUTISM SIBLING MAY BE the elephant in the room in autism adulthood. The brothers and sisters have grown up alongside autism and have had their entire lives shaped by its demands, limitations, and exciting growth. Yet most of the time, we are focused on how the parents feel, or how the autistic person himself feels. Parents write the books. Parents go to the conferences.

Parents also worry about the quality of life their children experience—all their children. They want each child to live as full a life as possible, but their autistic child requires a deeper, broader kind of planning. If that plan includes siblings, it is absolutely necessary that we look at their lives, their perspectives, and benefit from their ideas and resources.

One day soon I'd like to say to Max and Ben, "We're thinking of the future with your brother, but we'd like you to be part of this process; what kind of life do you want for your brother? Do you want him to be in the community? To have friends?" Max and Ben might decide, yeah, I can hang out with him a bit.

I don't think that Max and Ben think much at all about Nat's future and their role in it. I don't know, though. I am afraid to ask. What if they're really uncomfortable about the question; what if they shrug as if they don't care? Even though it is more likely that they'd feel, I am not ready to deal with what might be. So where do we start? How do we have this conversation with the siblings?

When a sibling is the guardian

I sought out siblings of older people with autism to learn what they went through, how their parents prepared them for whatever the future would be. Kara and Kristen are twenty-three-year-old twins who have a younger sister, Katie. The twins are Katie's standby guardians. Both Kristen and Kara are social workers, involved in the disability community. Kara is a graduate student working with children with disabilities, and she was gracious enough to talk to me at length about her experience as an adult autism sibling.

Kara and Kristen started a group called SIBS New Jersey to address the needs for siblings. "Our mom taught us before our sister was born to be accepting of disability," Kara said. "Mom taught us everyone is different; also that disability is very hard on the parent. We're a united front." Their mother talked to them about how it wasn't going to be easy because of what the outside world thought, but that as long as they stuck together, it would be OK. However, Kara was very quick to admit, "It's been an emotional roller coaster."

Kara told me a bit about how she first realized that she would one day be Katie's guardian, and how she dealt with the thought of this enormous responsibility. "I do remember when I was a senior in college two years ago, our parents told us they'd have to go through the process of making me her legal guardian—even though they are still alive. That's when it became real for me. I was devastated that I felt that I had a child already. It was one of the hardest things for me to go through. I was angry at all of them—very frustrated, confused. I dealt with it by saying, 'I have to do this; me and my sister are the only ones.' It became the reality. I had never fully realized this in high school. I finally acknowledged it."

At the time of this interview, Katie was attending a private school, funded by the school district—this had been the case for Nat, too. The Federal law (IDEA, Individuals with Disabilities Education Act) requires towns and cities to give every child a free and appropriate education, so if the child's team finds that the only appropriate setting is at an approved private school, the district pays for it.

In Katie's school, she learned most skills using Applied Behavioral Analysis (ABA), a popular autism approach that utilizes rewards as reinforcement for desired actions and behaviors. Katie's high school years have also consisted of community learning and occupational therapy. Her education, according to Kara, is "based in realism rather than in academics."

I asked Kara what challenges they have encountered so far in terms of Katie's care. "From an institutional standpoint," she said, "getting Katie an education and the services she needs. When I went to college and had to go away, I was very guilt-ridden leaving home. As a child you have to ask for what you need, but my parents already have so much on their plate. Yet somehow we've made it work."

Kara has not often felt comfortable with her interactions with the public when it comes to her sister's challenges. "I always wondered what people were going to think. Other families and extended family had not always been very understanding of disability. I figured I had to educate or ignore it—or burn myself out."

All special needs families need to think about what backups they have, what safety nets—both for their loved ones and for themselves. Kara said that being fiscally responsible is an important protective action. Getting the money right is absolutely paramount in managing the life of an adult with autism. Setting up a special needs trust—money that is not in the disabled person's name, but that is managed by another party—is a necessity. All autism families should seek the advice of an attorney who specializes in disability trusts, guardianships, and wills.

Kara and her family have taken care of Katie's finances, but the greater challenge is the less tangible question of supportive relationships to draw upon in case something happens to Kara or Kristen. She described her goals: "Educate my own future children, my sister's children. Continue this legacy of disability awareness. I want our kids to take care of things if need be. But there is no backup in terms of concrete plan, just do what we need to do and hope to God it works out."

Kara was quick to tell me that the resources available to siblings were scarce. She had to rely on her own strength and judgment to find her way with Katie's imminent adulthood. "Nothing, no resources, just innate resilience and coping. Having another sibling helped. I journal; I blog. I encourage others to find their art, music, writing, whatever you enjoy as your coping mechanism."

Kara felt that sibling networks on Facebook, the Internet, and in real life were the most helpful to her. She also praised the work of Don Meyer, an internationally renowned specialist in siblings and disability in the family (interviewed later in this chapter). Don created "Sibshops," workshops for siblings, which Kara felt were immensely helpful. "The Sibshop introduces siblings to ways of talking about their issues. They are therapeutic—not therapy. Activity-based. These were not available when I was growing up; Mom didn't have enough time to investigate for us."

To this end, she and her sister Kristen started SIBS New Jersey, just after attending a conference at Brandeis University entitled "Sibs Journey." Kara had found out about it through a siblings group on Facebook. "I met all these people; I always felt no one ever included us, it was always about the parents. Siblings are very rarely acknowledged or validated. I felt left out. I needed to talk to somebody, and didn't know anybody going through this. There's not a lot of support for the families going through the transition. The emotional aspect—there's not as much support as when the kids were younger."

Kara conferred with other grown siblings about what could be done to help others like them. They created SIBS NJ as a volunteer-run organization: "I thought that more than anything siblings need to network and form friendships and support one another. There's nothing like being able to share your experience with someone else who is going through what you're going through."

Kara's twin sister Kristen helps by offering her clinical experience as a social worker. Kristen organizes meetings and comes up with topics and presentations for parents. "She used to work in a division of an agency for people with Asperger's, on social skills. She now does behavioral work in group homes for people with intellectual disabilities and mental illness," said Kara, whose skill set is more about fundraising and development. She oversees social media and is the SIBS NJ president—the go-to person. She navigates funding and exposure.

Kara's advice to other families following in her footsteps was nothing surprising or magical, but absolutely true and inescapable:

"My parents were very good at explaining that I wouldn't be alone in this; they knew I could do it." Kara gives her parents credit especially in terms of their forthright attitude around Katie's disability and special needs. "You have to have the conversation. We have to approach the situation in a collaborative way and be honest. I was very happy because I was very much included. I was asked earlier in my life, 'Do you want to do that?' It comes with great responsibility and sacrifice. I think it was very fair."

Katie's imminent transition to adulthood weighs heavily on Kara. She wants her sister to have a worthwhile life. "She'll leave at twenty-one and hopefully she'll be in a day habilitation program. I would like her to have supported employment once a week."

Kara then laid out Katie's most likely living situation: "She'll live with our parents until they die. Or she'll live with me. I'll always need an extra bedroom. Eventually, within sixty-five years, she'll be in supported housing. But New Jersey is inundated, there is no housing in the state," Kara finished, making it clear that even when you painstakingly plan supports for an autistic loved one, there will still always be some uncertainties. Still, we plan, and we do our best. Living gracefully with that reality is probably the best we can do.

Growing up with an autistic sibling and loving it

I talked to Elijah, the son of my friend Kaija, whom I met years ago at an autism conference in South Dakota. Elijah was very forthcoming about his relationship with his autistic brother Aaron, who is eighteen. "His diagnosis is autism but it's FG syndrome—a rare genetic disorder which cause issues with growth, muscle mass, and digestive issues. But Aaron's got no particular diet; he eats chips, pudding, yogurt, and sandwiches. Diet has not necessarily had an impact on him, but I don't know for certain if we tried dietary restrictions."

Elijah does have other sibs: two half-sisters, Suzannah and Ellie.

"Aaron has the concept of family and what a brother is. We're very close. I see him once a week; I live fifty miles from Sioux Falls." He's a teenager, and doesn't want to hang out with his brother. "He says, 'bye bye.'" His vocabulary is limited, as are his social skills. Yet Elijah feels a "fairly strong" brotherly bond with Aaron:

I don't rough him up like most brothers do with each other. But still it's a healthy family relationship. He knows I don't take any of his shit. He's upstairs and asks "I want chips, I want DVD player"—Mom will get it for him, and I won't. I'll say "Go find your own DVD player, go get your own chips." When I come home, he wonders if I'll take care of him or if he has to work for himself. I am an institutor of helping him grow in his own way. He says, after ten seconds, "bye bye'" to me, which means "I need my own space."

Which is much like when Nat wants nothing to do with me and he says, "Mommy will go away."

Sometimes Elijah takes care of Aaron. "I'm currently at a school fifty miles away, but my first two years of college I spent in Sioux Falls, two blocks away. There was a part of me that made that decision because of Aaron, because if they needed assistance, I was there. They understood after my sophomore year when I made the decision to leave that school. They still know they can rely on me. Mom doesn't like to ask for help with Aaron. My dad is different, he's not afraid to say, 'Hey, I know you've got a big weekend planned, but could you come home for one night?'"

Elijah feels that his parents did the right thing, always making him feel like he had a choice about being a caregiver to Aaron. "They've never said, 'we need you to take care of Aaron.' The grand scheme of my own life has been my own choice. There was no direct moment in life when they brought it up, but through discussions like living wills, life insurance, the topic has come up a lot more. But, I never thought to myself, 'I will be Aaron's main caretaker in time.'"

Elijah seemed very healthy emotionally, very much his own person, who also knew how to look after his brother in his own way. "For me, Aaron's disability challenges are more like an obstacle in the obstacle course that you have to get over," explained Elijah. "In high school, I had a great friend group, but it always was a little strange to tell them, 'Hey this is my brother, he has autism, he's not going to be able to communicate with you like you expect.'" However, Elijah told me with grave seriousness that he wouldn't be friends with people who didn't get that. He told people his brother was a little different but was still a fun guy. "He's going to shake your hand and tell you that you have nice hair. His emotions do shift. When we go out to eat, he wants to shake all the waitresses' hands and tell them they're pretty. It's what we know; it's sort of the norm."

Aaron is currently a high school sophomore, and spends his time in resource rooms. Elijah does not think much of the education Aaron is getting. "I'm not 100 percent sure what he's learning—they send stuff home that he's colored; it's not that legible." This sparked an old feeling of annoyance in me—the way some school systems still do not focus enough on pragmatics. Elijah reasoned, "Preparing him for the real world is not quite an option anymore. We all realize it's going to be difficult for him to have a real world job at twenty-three. He doesn't have the vocabulary or ability to make his way. We want to teach him to make his own food, communicate with others, tell people what his name is. The school is working toward allowing him to be his own person in society. He has educational assistance there; from kindergarten through fifth grade he had a direct educational aide, paid for by the city. She would also take care of him outside of school—that was paid for out of my parents' pocket and the city as well." This is a common arrangement, I have found. Many times we hired Nat's aides and teachers to come over and supplement his skills after school. Sometimes, but not often, the school system paid for after-school help.

Elijah told me all this without any bitterness, an attitude he comes by perhaps just by being a guy of twenty-one. Or perhaps he really is facing reality and taking it from there. I could learn a lot from Elijah, I think.

Elijah was a little bit unsure about Aaron's future after twenty-two. "In the near future, I presume he will stay with my parents. They're very uncertain as to what his living situation will be. In Sioux Falls there's not a lot. There are some group homes, we would try to find some group, a community of three to four other men he would stay with, people watching over him; most likely in six to seven years we will have to design ourselves some sort of group facility, because there's not anything."

Elijah does not often think about Aaron's future and his role in it. To be honest, I can't imagine why any young man would want to, because they are young and they haven't yet fully imagined their own futures, let alone a disabled brother's. Elijah reminded me of Max when he said, "I don't process things that way; I think of a year from now, a day at a time. It's incredibly likely that I will be not his caretaker, but rather, his primary source. I don't know what that will entail. That's the bridge we'll come to. For my own perspective, our family life is great, I love my mom and dad, my siblings. There hasn't been much tension. I trust them. Yes, at this moment I don't know twenty years from now what the situation will be, but I know that because of how my parents have handled the matter our entire lives, that they will be able to communicate what they will like from me. I know that they'll give us a path to follow once they're gone."

But why couldn't he share this responsibility with his half-sisters? "I couldn't say," he said, and did not care to elaborate on that. It may be that in Elijah's life, it has been his parents' openness and honesty that have informed him the most, and made him feel safe and important in his own right. And that's not necessarily a job for one's siblings, in the natural order of things. Though I have to say that I am always grateful, relieved—that it actually takes my breath away when I see Max and Ben taking care of each other, when I see their love and kindness for each other.

Other than his parents' support, Elijah hasn't found any particularly helpful resource with regard to life with his autistic brother: "None in particular. It is a day-to-day struggle, not a major effect on me emotionally. Yes, he's different, yes, there are major challenging aspects to it. All in all, I never knew anything different. I never had a younger brother who is 'normal.' It's never been that much of an issue, because it's never been any other way. Mine is just a little more different." Similarly, Max and Ben are fond of repeating Nat's odd, charming words, "It's a different, that's OK."

An older sib, a very different worldview

My sibling research took me to some older siblings in their fifties and sixties. Pamela from South Carolina and her younger sister Sheila are from a completely different era than Nat, Katie, or Aaron. Sheila, who is fifty-six, is "like a five-year-old," Pamela said. The incident that led to her institutionalization was something right out of the movie *Rain Man*. When they were children, Pamela's mother discovered Sheila and her two-year-old sister trying to stuff a blanket into an electric heater. Their mother's fear and horror led her to institutionalize Sheila at seven years old. I know *Rain Man* is not a real story, but it certainly has a lot of truth in it—even to me, a modern-era mom. Pamela confirmed that.

Currently, Sheila lives in a program north of Worcester, Massachusetts. "It looks like a small college," said Pamela. "Most of its programs are for school-aged children. They have apartments in Clinton, probably four apartments with four people in them, and the house she's in has another three. This adult service part probably has thirty or so people. They have another ten in a small assisted living program. The provider has done a good job of adapting to the changes in standards, and so now the vast majority of their business is short-term intensive schooling. They have stayed loyal to their older adult group; ten years ago they moved to apartments in the community."

Nationwide, most institutions are going through this sort of transition, or closing down. When you hear the stories about the old institutions, you imagine that there was not one positive thing about them. But Pamela was telling me something very different: Sheila has mostly lived in one branch or another of her current program for decades. Pamela feels they have been good to her.

Perhaps some of these institutions had enough wise and humane people at the helm that they were able to transition to becoming modern residential schools—like the one Nat attended. Pamela is very glad that Sheila's place has not closed down but rather has adapted to the times. Pamela has observed how comfortable Sheila has been there all these years, and she attributes this in part to the stability of staffing: "A number of the staff have been there ten years or more. She has a friendly relationship with the staff and co-residents. The Director of Adult Services has been there twenty years. I think the institution has a commitment to their residents, and probably how they treat their staff, though I don't know much about that. I have a sense of their long-term commitment to their residents."

All of Pamela's life, even though Sheila did not live at home for most of it, she tried hard to be "the easy one" for her parents. "I grew up to be a very responsible kid and person, even though my parents tried to protect me from feeling responsible, and they encouraged me to live my own life. Still, growing up, I was under pressure to be the good kid, to not be any trouble." Pam did not feel that her parents did much to foster the siblings' relationship: "My mother felt like this was the great tragedy of her life. I never understood that. I felt that Sheila was happy; it seemed like a good way to live, not really concerned about the past or future."

About ten years ago, Pamela's mother sent her an email describing what she wanted when she could no longer take care of Sheila: "Send birthday cards, Christmas presents; have her visit the family summer home, which she loves." Her mother probably had many such thoughts about Sheila's distant future, but didn't share them all with Pam.

Pam said, "I have one memory of going to the institution as a child—and hoping they didn't think I lived there. I was more comfortable with having Sheila come home." And even though Sheila didn't live at home, throughout Pam's childhood, she was part of the family for Christmas, Easter, and summer. "In my thirties, I went home for Easter, and Sheila was home. I said I'd take her to church, because she loves church and Mother didn't. Sheila loved to say the Lord's Prayer. She says it fairly loudly and slowly. But when people turned around, they smiled at her. She has some of the facial features of an intellectually disabled person; she looks cognitively disabled even though she doesn't have Down's syndrome. This is the way the world should be: she should be able to go to church and have people smile at her."

Pamela and Sheila have two younger half-sisters, one of whom is taking primary responsibility for their mother, who for the last three or four years has begun to have symptoms of Alzheimer's disease. Their grandmother died of Alzheimer's, and so when Pam and her sisters saw the initial signs of forgetfulness in their mother, "we took it very seriously." And so, in early 2012, Pam started to take primary responsibility of Sheila and went through the process of becoming her legal guardian. "I'm good at organizing, at figuring things out, managing details. I'm less the warm fuzzy one. I really see it as they [the institution] are her family, too."

Pam manages to do a lot for Sheila all the way from her home in South Carolina, partially by using a special consultant she hired from Arc of Massachusetts. Some of Pamela's biggest concerns as Sheila's caregiver and guardian as she ages are about changes and restrictions in the laws: "My concern is that the laws for assisted living limits the things they can do. Massachusetts has strict laws about putting someone with developmental delay in a nursing home. A guardian cannot make the decision to put someone in long term, although the court can make that decision." The state is worried about people being warehoused, which, of course, is an understandable fear.

Pamela has direct experience with the strict and sometimes rigid and unaccommodating laws: "Sheila broke her ankle in the beginning of June 2014 and had to have surgery, had to go to a nursing home. The doctor could not schedule surgery for a week, the hospital said she didn't need to be there, and the group home couldn't take her if she needed two staff to move her from the wheelchair. The nursing homes couldn't take her partly because of the legal complications!"

Pamela began to realize fairly recently that Sheila's provider was not as competent in terms of legal issues as she had assumed. Even though Pamela feels that the staff knows her sister better than she does, she began to understand that she would have to take a more active fiduciary and legal role in her sister's life. "I was doing research about nursing home issues and came upon the Arc of Massachusetts's consulting branch. You can get one of the consultants to evaluate your sibling at a transition point. I signed up and I was very pleased. The consultant was very impressed by the program where Sheila lives, and how thoughtful the staff were."

When Pamela became Sheila's guardian, the program recommended a lawyer who had a special needs law practice. Pam's father was an executive, and loved managing his money, but had made some significant mistakes because he had used a lawyer who didn't specialize in special needs law or finance. He had created a trust for her sister, but the wrong kind of trust. He gave Sheila an equal number of shares in the summer house, which were in her name, not in the trust. This would mean she had assets, which would then likely endanger any possible benefits from government sources. So after Pam became guardian, she had to remedy some of this. Sheila is getting her funding through DDS now.

"I realized from the incident with the nursing home that I had to update my understanding. My sense of Sheila's life was mostly from my early childhood and early adulthood. My understanding of how people like Sheila can have the best life has changed so much. That led to the insight of why the court doesn't trust guardians: the guardians' thinking might be outdated. I realized I really had to keep researching. I can trust Sheila's program, but I have to keep researching what the best practices are now. I do feel good about it. I feel a little bit that you might judge me because I'm from such a different world. But keeping updated is one of the keys."

Me? Judge her? On the contrary, I'm in awe of her. To bridge the two eras with the grace and success that Pam has is something I can only imagine.

Pamela recommended that people in need of help or advice in caring for an adult with autism should look into the large service providers or advocacy groups: "Any larger organization or service provider is going to have a social worker. Use their social worker. Those who can't afford to consult with a disabilities lawyer or hire private consultants need to push to have those social workers sit down with them, talk to them about long-term planning, quality of life, choices for day habilitation or supported job programs. Push the social workers. It should be their job."

You have to ask for help, Pamela reminds us. For Pam's own peace of mind, it was important to discover other adult siblings going through the same thing she was. "I joined a sib group on Facebook. Some siblings were still home with parents until parents could no longer keep them, and then they took them into their home." This is just what I had found that Kara is planning to do for her disabled sibling, Katie. But in Pamela's case, Sheila truly *is* an adult. She didn't like the same things that moved her as a child. She has an IQ of around thirty, with seizures that can't be fully controlled, yet she has a sense of herself.

Pam said, "I want family members to be the ones figuring out what's best for her. That's not always possible, but it ought to be that way in general. A balance is best in spreading the work around: having professionals who decide, and families who can take it on. I'm lucky my kids got to college age before I became guardian," she added.

As in Nat's and my case, Pamela can understand Sheila somewhat. Probably many caregivers know that the way to communicate with their client or loved one is to frame questions that can be easily answered. Like Nat, Sheila's ability to understand is well above her ability to communicate.

The staff can understand Sheila's speech better than Pam can, which makes Pam very happy—we always want our loved ones' caregivers to really "get them." Recently, they told Pamela that Sheila had said that "her foot is tingling," an impressive bit of detail for Sheila to verbalize.

Sibshops: offering critical support for the brothers and sisters

"Anything you could say about being the parent of children with special needs (mental health, etc.), you could pretty much say the same about brothers and sisters," Don Meyer said to me in a phone interview. "They're going to have many—if not most—of the issues that parents have, in addition some of their own. However, in terms of attention paid to their needs, the siblings are getting the short end of the stick."

These brothers and sisters will likely have the longest lasting relationship; at least longer than a service provider, and possibly longer than the parents. "Over the long haul no one logs on more hours than brothers and sisters," said Don. "In the end, it's going to be the brothers and sisters, not the parents, who come through, and they need help to succeed in this role, they need support for themselves."

Don's project, Sibshops, has been a very productive and successful venture, providing young brothers and sisters the supports that parents get. Sibshops provide a forum to connect with someone walking down a similar path, as well as a way of learning coping skills through the group dynamic. Don has also created online groups like SibTeen as well as one for adults called SibNet.

Don has found that it is the sisters who carry the burden of care most of the time: "SibNet is about 97 percent sisters, as sibling issues are in lot of ways sister issues. Typically a new SibNet member is a sister in her forties with an autistic sibling. She needs information, validation, support; the most sought-after are the latter two benefits." At the Sibshops sessions and online forums, Don has observed that it is not always solutions the siblings need; some just want to be heard: "Some present incredibly problematic situations and scenarios. The others online will chime in and say, 'I hear you, I have the same issue with my sister, my brother,' and that same kid who presented the knotty problem is writing back saying, 'I feel so much better, thank you.' The same problem is still there, but she feels better because she's been heard."

Forty years is a long time to wait for validation.

Of course siblings should get their help much sooner than that, but you can't always get young people to go do that. "It's incumbent upon the people running the Sibshops to make the sessions rewarding on many levels. They serve fun food and play games so that members want to come back, even if they've had their arm twisted to go the first time," Don said. In our case, Max was willing to go to a support group at Nat's school when he was little, but Ben was another story. He would not go; I was even afraid to ask him. I didn't want his life to be about autism, even if it meant taking care of himself around the autism. I never got past seeing that I'd have to twist Ben's arm, so I never sent him. This was my own decision—one that I still question. All I can say is that I did the best I could at the time.

Don has found that siblings want to know how their parents have planned for the future. They also need to know that they have a choice as to how involved they want to be. "Let them know there's a range of options for helping. Many feel they have far fewer degrees of freedom," Don told me. The truth is that brothers and sisters actually think at a very early age about the days to come, so parents need to be aware of this and accommodate it as early as possible. "I hear frustration when the parents won't talk about the future," Don said.

Don recommends that parents keep an open conversation as the kids grow up. "Give kids opportunities commensurate with other kids their age, they'll benefit . . . whether backpacking through Europe or whatever . . . they will feel like they have a life of their own. I don't think you can begin it too early, a casual discussion even. 'Someday Tim may be living on his own, we're all trying to work toward making it successful so that Tim can live in the community . . .'"

When the sibling matures and is more ready to hear specifics, then parents can discuss things like guardianship, or goals and wishes for the disabled sibling. But until then, the siblings may not be ready to handle such details.

"I had one seventeen-year-old girl speak with tears in her eyes about the plans she had for her brother: 'My sister and I will buy a house together. Neither of us will get married and one will work during the day and the other during the night,'" To live under the assumption that you will be so tied to your sibling that you won't marry or live without him or have a particular kind of job—this is sad and unfair. It is stunting that child's growth.

If the parents make the effort to open up the conversations much earlier in their typical child's life, and to free them to be their own people with their own dreams, the outcome will likely be positive for all. "Chances are those sibs are going to be involved. They're going to have the longest lasting relationship, after all. I tell people, if you don't want to attend to typically developing sibs, do so anyway for their disabled brothers and sisters! It's easy to make an argument that if you want to assure a good long-term outcome for people with disabilities, you should invest in their brothers and sisters," Don advised.

Parents, of course, need to be incredibly proactive about the plans for the future of the special needs kid. None of us want to have to work so hard, nor to think so starkly about the future, but we need to do this for our children—all of them. Don said, "Parents and service providers need to engage in reflective listening. What this means is that you're not solving the problem, you're not explaining, you're just *reflecting* on it." Parents need to hear their typically developing kids, and to hear that this is not easy. First and foremost, a parent must take care of his children, and the special needs child should not have the primary spot of concern all the time. There has to be balance. No sibling signed up for this role. As obvious as this might be, it is important to remember that each sibling is a person in their own right—not a keeper. Don said, "There are a lot of kids who grow up with a 'job description.' How many of us would like that?"

The number one point, to Don, is a right to one's own life. Self-determination is for *everybody.* "I think if we support, inform, validate, and celebrate brothers and sisters as they grow up, they will elect to be involved in the lives of the siblings who have disabilities when their parents no longer can . . . I think siblings should be given some degrees of freedom as they grow up." If allowed to have their own lives, the vast majority of them will likely step up to the plate of their own accord and be involved with their disabled sibling later in life.

A different kind of sibling

Once Nat moved into his apartment with John, I was able to sit back in satisfaction for the first time in Nat's adulthood. We had clearly done the right thing. Nat appeared relaxed with his new routine and place very quickly. One thing that did worry me was that he was losing weight, despite everyone's best efforts. I ultimately took him to a prominent gastrointestinal specialist whose research was primarily with autistic people. We learned that Nat was lactose intolerant, had significant acid reflux, and also had some esophagitis. He was put on omeprazole, which helped tremendously. According to many autism specialists, around one-third of the people with autism have some sort of GI issue that should be looked into and that frequently account for difficult behaviors like self-injury.

A few months into Nat's transition to city life, John took a second job as the manager of a day program because he wanted more experience in the field of disability. I felt some anxiety over this change because I wondered if it signaled a desire for John to move on from such intensive caregiving.

But John assured me this was not the case: "Nat is my little brother," he said. "I am always going to be a part of his life." My insides started to melt at that. Nat was indeed in good hands, with someone who loved him. However, John had his own needs; he had a lot of ambition and drive, and he needed the challenge of the additional job. Even though Nat usually came home to live with us on the weekends, John required more respite for his own life's demands. And even if that meant a bit more demand on us, we liked the fact that John was so multifaceted and driven. John was not simply "phoning it in" with Nat; he was trying to build a rich and layered life for *both* of them.

Still, the shared living arrangement requires that the caregiver makes the client his top priority. The shared living provider is responsible for the client 24/7—not the parents or guardian. And while the parents or guardian have the ultimate decision-making power over the important aspects of their child's entire life, the caregiver is the first line of oversight and protection.

Nat was indeed John's top priority. And yet, if John followed his career path, taking graduate school courses and other jobs in the field, it meant that he could not always be there when Nat got home from his day program. Clearly John would need a respite worker for certain weekdays, so that Nat would have seamless supervision. I felt nervous at the thought of a new guy coming in and working with Nat, but John already knew someone good who was available. "Besides," John told me, "Nat has already met him, because he has come by to hang out sometimes." *Hmm, really?* I thought, not sure how I felt about that, this stranger spending time with Nat, someone I didn't even know. But then I realized Nat was a twenty-four-year-old man and was becoming more independent of us. Meeting new people was part of growing up. And I would have to become more independent, too—of Nat. I would have to trust John and trust Nat. And that is how Danny came into our lives.

When John first told me about Danny, he described him as "the exact opposite of me. Plays sports, more masculine, calmer . . ." He said all this laughing. By this point, John and I had a very easygoing relationship. There's no other way I could let Nat live with someone I had never met. I would have to trust and be completely comfortable with the caregiver or else forget the whole thing.

Danny was close to Nat's age, like John. He was a big friendly teddy bear of a guy, bearded and bright-eyed. I liked him right away. He showed up at Nat's birthday party, which was at one of those indoor trampoline places. Several of Nat's friends already knew Danny because he had been a staff person at one of the other group homes run by our service provider.

I loved the way he was such a good sport, jumping with the guys and then coming back for cake at our house. It was all a little awkward, the way birthday parties can be, because the parents/caregivers don't always know what to do with themselves and they sometimes don't even eat the cake. So we did a bit of just sitting around the dining room table watching Nat and his friends stuff cake in their mouths and look around for seconds.

Soon after Nat's birthday party, we decided to have a little evening Chanukah celebration, and on impulse I invited Danny and John. I felt like it might be a nice thing to get to know Danny better, but to be honest, dinner parties are hard for me, much like birthday parties. But John accepted right away, saying he loves my brisket—which already made the whole thing feel easier.

They came in and just like John always had, Danny made himself at home. They joked with each other and Nat in front of us, which was a good way to get us all to relax. I offered them wine, and pretty soon we were all laughing around the table, including Ben, and talking about piercings and tattoos (I had just gotten a tattoo on my side, which really impressed Danny). Ben probably felt like Danny was cool enough to "chill" with, and so we all ate and joked. After the dinner we went into the living room to hang out a little more. Danny and John squeezed into the chair-and-a-half, which was a little odd, but silly and sweet, too. Their easy laughter and gentle teasing of each other made the night truly fun, and not at all a burden. And just like that, Nat now had *two* older brothers.

Online Resources

- "Managing someone else's money," an article by Naomi Karp in *Consumer Finance Protection Bureau*—this is a guide that will help sibling or parent autism guardians and caregivers with the financial issues of taking care of an autistic person: www.consumerfinance.gov/blog/managing-someone-elses-money/
- Sibteen FB group offers validation, story-sharing, emotional support: www.facebook.com/groups/SibTeen/
- If there isn't a Sibshop for their age, teens can volunteer at a Sibshop for younger kids, as a mentor. They may be able to earn service learning hours from their high school (go to the Sibshop tab and find a state by state listing) https://www.siblingsupport.org/sibshops.
- Join a group like the Sibling Leadership Network. These guys step in, even when their parents are still involved: www.siblingleadership.org
- Organization for Autism Research's Sibling Support Initiative: www.researchautism.org/family/familysupport/SiblingSupportInitiative.asp

Books

- *Families, Illness and Disability: an Integrative Treatment Model*, John S. Rolland (Basic Books, 1994)
- *How to Talk so Kids will Listen & Listen so Kids Will Talk*, Elaine Mazlish and Adele Faber (Scribner, 2012)
- *Special Siblings: Growing Up with Someone with a Disability*, Mary McHugh (Brookes Publishing, 2002)
- *Sibling Survival Guide*, edited by Don Meyer and Emily Holl (Woodbine House, 2014)
- *The Normal One*, Jeanne Safer (Delta, 2003)
- *Being the Other One*, Kate Strohm (Shambhala, 2005)
- *The Ride Together*, Paul Karasik and Judy Karasik (Washington Square Press, 2004)
- *Hamlet's Dresser*, Bob Smith (Scribner, 2003)

Chapter Nine:

AUTISM ADULTHOOD HEALTH AND SAFETY ISSUES

Figuring out if he's safe

The summer that Nat turned twenty-five, our lives changed in a completely different, unexpected direction: a new health issue. I think I started noticing something was happening with Nat in September of that year. I got a call just as I was parking, about to meet a friend for coffee. It was from Richard, the day program director. Richard got right to it: "I don't know how to tell you this. But Nat came in with puffy eyes and was really not himself, you know the way he's been lately." A poisonous feeling started flooding my throat. Oh, I knew.

Richard continued, "He was hanging his head, quiet, not talking to himself, not walking around. I asked him some questions—he started crying a little."

"What questions?" I broke in, wanting to cry myself. But I already kind of knew. Richard had asked Nat questions about whether someone had been touching him, hurting him. At the time this was all we could imagine because he had seemed healthy, and he had adjusted well to his apartment living with John. Nevertheless, Nat had not been himself for a while. He'd been so still. So quiet. And where did I go with that? The worst place possible: worrying that he'd been abused. This is not a frivolous fear, either. I know cases of such abuse. Moreover, the Center for Disease Control reports that "one in six boys are sexually abused at one time or another, and the numbers for individuals with disabilities are even higher."

Richard told me that he'd asked Nat if something hurt. Nat had gestured to his abdomen, but Richard thought Nat's hands were pointing kind of close to his crotch. Richard asked him some more stuff like, "Did someone hurt you?" and Nat answered, "Yes."

One part of my brain just froze. I tried to grab hold of my thoughts, but they had formed a dense cloud in my head. I needed to get off the phone. I needed to think. I needed to figure this out. I called Ned, expecting him to be Mr. Rational as always, to organize my thoughts, tell me not to worry. But for once he was just as hesitant as I was. "What are we supposed to do?" he kept asking. "I don't know," I kept answering. "There's going to be an investigation, of everyone Nat spends time with. I don't know," I said, book-ending my uncertainty.

I drove home, but I didn't get out of the car. I just sat there, in my driveway, screaming, "Oh Nat!" and then, "I'm sorry, Nat. No. No way. God, please. No." My throat got raw. I drove to the day program. I didn't get out the car right away; instead, I called Nat's doctor. I love his doctor. She's a Jewish mother, just like me. She's known Nat forever. She sounded like she was crying when I told her. She asked to be kept in the loop. But what was the loop? Right now it was all a knot.

When I finally got hold of Nat, he was very warm. The heat from his skin was like a heavy blanket. His eyes were not the usual crystal blue. They were a hot Bermudan blue. He was sick. No one had realized this, though. I drove him home.

I asked him in different ways if he was happy, if he was hurt. I asked him what hurt. Where did it hurt, who'd hurt him? But of course it was so hard to get any reliable information. The conversation went like this:

"Does your head hurt?"

"Head. Yes."

"Do your feet hurt?"

"Yes. Feet."

Sigh. True? Or just the default answer? "Nat: does the chair hurt?"

"Yes." Talking is truly the most difficult thing you can ask of Nat.

Not once did I get an answer that was anything like a confirmation of abuse. Finally I asked him about if anyone touched his private parts.

"No."

No. Two letters. So definite. So rare with Nat. But with Nat, unlike his "yes," "no" means no.

A cool wave of relief swept over me. My thoughts cleared for the first time that day: Nat was sick.

I gave him Tylenol. He went to sit in the big yellow armchair, in the sunny bay window. I checked on him, while sending around an email update to his whole team that I believed he was actually sick, and not sad. Not hurt.

And then, I thought I saw the flash of teeth. Then, his voice bubbled up: a small curve of laughter. Laughter. Oh God, how beautiful.

Using my intuition

But the fever still bothered me. And the dark, silent mood he'd been in that had led Richard to such a dire conclusion. I realized that he was indeed gesturing at his abdomen. The right side. *Wait, where is the appendix?* Another call to the doctor, and there we were, in the emergency room. We told the doctors there about everything, even the allegation of abuse. They examined Nat thoroughly. At one point Nat giggled at the doctor's palpations.

He was no longer quiet or still. Whatever it was, it had passed. By now, my husband and I were feeling a bit like overly anxious newbie parents. But of course we had to check things out with someone who is practically nonverbal. I will always be that over-anxious mother.

An ultrasound and many blood tests later, Nat was deemed fine but gassy. Exhausted, we took Nat home. Our best guess? Some kind of benign virus.

A new diagnosis

We thought we were out of the woods in terms of illness or abuse. But we still noticed that half the time he'd come home for the weekends with his light out. I stored away my worry and redoubled my efforts to make him smile, doing his favorite things with him: bike rides, long walks, Facebook messaging with my family.

But eventually, by June it became clear that something scary and new was indeed happening. We were at the Harvard University pool, for the Special Olympics State Games, when Nat's team began their relay. At either side of the pool stood teammates waiting to jump in for their turn.

Nat was up third. The second swimmer approached him, and he stood alert, waiting. When it was time, his body curved into an arch, ready to dive.

But there he remained. He just stood there, poised over the lip of the pool, not moving.

What is going on? "Nat, go!" I yelled.

Still no dive. I yelled again. And again. I tried to walk closer to where he was standing, but I was blocked by a lot of people and a plexiglass-topped wall. Ned joined in with me shouting at Nat, trying to get his attention. We screamed ourselves hoarse. "I guess it's because he has a different coach over there," said Ned, trying to figure it out. "She doesn't know to tell him firmly to get in the water." My anger shot way up. Why would they do that? Why would they give him a different coach!? Didn't they know how much he needed routines to stay the same?

But—*was* it the coach? Or something else? A new unnamed fear unfurled inside. "NAT! GET IN!" I willed him to get the f*** in that pool. This was SOMA State Games, Nat's favorite day of the year. Why wouldn't he move?

Finally, after what seemed like hours, and after the race was long over, Nat went in. He swam great. Everyone in the stadium clapped.

But this was not over. I had to face it: the odd hesitation, the immovable silence had been happening since perhaps September. Nat would come home some weekends as if in a daze. No smiles, no stimming, no pacing, no thumb-sucking. No self-talk. Just standing or sitting very still, arms drawn out in front of him, his lips drawn tightly over his teeth as if someone had said, "Nat! Close your mouth!"

So for months I had been worrying that someone somewhere was being mean to him, abusive, and that his spirit was being crushed. I kept asking him, in ways I thought he'd understand, "Is someone being bad to Nat? Are you hurt? Do you like your job?" Peppering him with all sorts of useless questions, just indulging my panic. Nat can't usually answer those sort of questions accurately. I don't know where the sentences I shoot at him go; I imagine lances falling impotently as they hit his kryptonite skull. Except Nat is the good guy.

During this time, Nat would also have bizarre outbursts of hysterical laughter. This was occurring everywhere—at home, in restaurants, on the job—and it was very difficult for any of us to control.

It seemed like there was no middle ground for Nat's behavior or emotions anymore. I began thinking back over the year. I had a new take on the episode I described above, when Richard had called us, and how strange Nat had been acting, and how we attributed it all to a fever in the end. Had that really been the complete explanation of what was happening to Nat? Now, six months since that September, he had no fever.

What was it, then? Seizures? Depression? Bipolar? And what about abuse? But we'd been over that one. I actually felt fairly confident that had it been abuse, he would not be able to laugh at other times. Or willingly go back to his routines of living with his caregiver and going to his day program.

Off to the doctors. Several different specialists later, we ended up with our neurologist of twenty-two years—Dr. Bauman, a pioneer in autism research, a tireless caring doctor and brilliant neurologist from the Integrated Center for Child Development in Newton. She watched a brief video Ned had taken of Quiet Nat, and she said, "This is not seizures. This is not depression. This looks like catatonia to me."

What was that? "Catatonia. This is a small subtype of autism. It means he freezes up. He literally can't move himself forward. Can't do the simplest things at the moment he's experiencing it." She added, "In 2006, Dr. Lorna Wing was one of the first to bring the issue of catatonia to the attention of the medical world [in her article "A Systematic Examination of Catatonia-like Clinical Pictures in Autism Spectrum Disorders," in *International Review of Neurobiology*]. Unfortunately, I don't think much has changed with regard to our understanding of the 'disorder' since that time. We may be hearing more about it because health care professionals are more aware of its existence."

I did some digging that night. On the National Institute of Health website, I came across a 2014 *Frontiers in Psychiatry* article called "Decalogue of Catatonia in Autism Spectrum Disorders" by Dirk M. Dhossche that began with a serious, if not downright dramatic, plea for more attention to catatonia from the scientific community: "This article is an unabashed drum roll for increased recognition and treatment of catatonia in autism spectrum disorders." Catatonia is defined in *Frontiers in Psychiatry* as a severe but treatable syndrome that warrants prompt diagnosis and treatment with benzodiazepines and electroconvulsive therapy (ECT) and that occurs in patients of all ages, including children and adolescents. The syndrome becomes critical and life threatening in its malignant form when aggravated by fever and autonomic dysfunction. Advances in catatonia research have segued into the field of autism over the last ten years. Catatonia in ASD has been increasingly recognized at a rate of 4–17 percent in adolescents and adults with ASD. No systematic studies have been done in preadolescent and older (>60 years old) patients.

That last sentence is what makes my blood boil. Where is the "autism awareness" for our guys, the older, more involved autistics?

There in Dr. Bauman's office, I was barely able to marshal my thoughts but I did manage to ask, "What do we do?" This was starting to feel horribly familiar, a nightmarish deja vu to those early days of Nat's diagnosis. In a blog post around this time I wrote, "I didn't get to just stick my toe into this river of pain, and test its temperature. No, I fell in, completely, this Thursday afternoon, when our doctor told us that she thinks Nat has something called 'autism catatonia.' It was a cruel flashback to 1993 when Nat was three, first diagnosed with autism. And here we were, with the very same doctor."

But in Nat's case, now, as a possibly catatonic autistic adult, Dr. Bauman felt she was not an expert in this area—I disagree; to me the sun rises and sets with Dr. B.—because she is a child neurologist. Yet she sees young adults on the spectrum because they have few other options for adult specialists. Dr. B. told us that she had recently come across several young men with the same symptoms as Nat. She wanted us to see one of two specialists in the country whom she felt were more experienced with catatonia. One was in California, one in New York.

We had an appointment with the New York specialist, which the doctor canceled, telling us that Nat was too old for his practice. He referred us to another specialist, who told us the same thing. Our failure to see these specialists, due to Nat being an adult, added another layer of frustration to our search for help.

Dr. Bauman had warned us that this might happen: as I have found from the loneliness of Nat's twenty-five years of life, the world is only now becoming competent in autism childhood. And despite twenty-five-plus years of the Americans with Disabilities Act, there does seem to be a degree of invisibility of adults with full-blown autism to the rest of society. My friend Robin, whom I interviewed for the Housing Chapter, has frequently asked me, rhetorically, "Where are all the autistic adults? Where are all the older ones?"

But similar to what Dr. Seuss's Horton the Elephant found, when he tried to show everyone his microscopic Who friends, the greater community seems a bit blind to our cries. And yet: we are here, we are here. We are here. And we need more specialists to help us when our loved ones cannot help themselves.

The blogging I did at that time is raw with pain:

I tried to be strong. I was simply going to learn about this condition of Nat's. Right away. I was not my thirty-year-old self, after all, caught in a hurricane of ignorance and fear. I am not going to be sad, I told people. What good would that do? But when you fall into that river, you can't simply get out. And that's where I am. Wet, cold, tired. It's not a rational thing, pain. It just happens. Your child is sick, you're sick. You can't bear what he might be feeling. You are him, but you're also not.

Silly me, I thought that we were full steam ahead into autism adulthood and that my main concerns now would be making sure Nat enjoyed his life—his job, his apartment, his activities in the evenings and weekends. It's been a pleasure watching him move into adulthood with such ease. I look back now and I see that it has gone really smoothly, even with all the housing issues we encountered. For the bottom line is that Nat has always had people around him who love him and also really like him, and he just thrives in that kind of light.

But something new, something evil has crept into his neurons—his long, curly, clumped, glorious neurons, that had always

*grown the way they wanted to, not according to the typical. As
I type this, my chest tightens and the tears start again. My eyes
already burn and are gray around the sockets. So much crying, in
just two days of being on the island of Catatonia.*

    I'm so scared.

Dr. Bauman scheduled a series of metabolic-analysis blood
and urine tests to rule out metabolic disorders associated with
autism, such as mitochondrial diseases, which according to the
Center for Disease Control are when "the mitochondria [in
one's cells] cannot efficiently turn sugar and oxygen into energy,
so the cells do not work correctly." The tests were also to determine if he had an autoimmune deficiency. Additionally, we
were asked for a complete medical history, and asked about any
genetic testing Nat had had. Years back we had tested Nat for
Fragile X Syndrome, which is often associated with autism, and
defined by the National Institute of Health as "a genetic condition that causes a range of developmental problems including
learning disabilities and cognitive impairment." But we would
have to rule out the others.

In the meantime, we set up an appointment for an electroen-
cephalogram (EEG) to rule out brain seizures. That test turned
out normal, though we were cautioned that the test is really a
snapshot only of the brain activity in that particular hour when
the test is taken. The final test Nat would have was a cranial MRI.

Meanwhile, I was doing my own research, mostly talking to
other autism parents whose autistic children had developed similar symptoms in adulthood. Three of these moms described their
child's version of autism catatonia. But as the first of these moth-
ers spoke, I found myself feeling that her descriptions did not
match what was going on with Nat at all. Only the fourth mom's
story felt at all like ours.

She told me that her son had been experiencing mood
swings—anger and the giddiness—and was ultimately diagnosed
with bipolar disorder. I learned that the meds used were extremely

effective in helping alleviate her son's symptoms. Her description of her son's erratic, up-and-down behavior resonated with me, with what I was observing in Nat. Also, importantly, I have the diagnosis of mild bipolar, also known as mood disorder. And there are many neurological anxiety-type disorders in my family besides. So I began wondering if what we were seeing was bipolar, and not a movement disorder like catatonia.

Next we went to see Dr. Christopher McDougle, Professor of Psychiatry and Pediatrics at the Massachusetts General Hospital and the MassGeneral Hospital for Children, who is also the director and a leading psychopharmacologist at the Lurie Center, a new complex associated with MassGeneral, which was dedicated to taking care of people on the spectrum for the entire lifespan. Finally, specialists with experience treating adults! A rare commodity indeed.

This doctor believed Nat was experiencing depression and mood swings, which resonated with me. We started Nat on a trial of Tegretol, reporting by email to the doctor every week on progress. Nat seemed to be less still, and not as silly in the weeks that followed. We felt cautiously relieved that perhaps we had found an answer.

I corresponded with Dr. McDougle over the next few months, discussing Nat's progress and also learning more about the state of adult autistic medical issues as he saw it. He wrote:

One of the biggest concerns is simply identifying primary care physicians who will care for adults with autism. Most physicians who care for adults have never seen an adult with autism for a routine medical check-up or a specific medical problem. When they were in medical school and during their residency training, they were unlikely to have been taught how to do a physical examination or treat an adult with autism. Until this hurdle can be overcome, it would be helpful if pediatricians providing medical care for individuals with autism would continue to care for these patients for a longer period of time than they usually do for their more typical patients.

I asked Dr. McDougle to list some of the main health concerns one might come across in autism adulthood:

As far as specific health concerns, the emergence of seizures in late adolescence/early adulthood is one to be aware of. In autism, there are two primary peaks of seizure onset, very early in life and then again in late adolescence/early adulthood.

Another health concern would be gastroesophageal reflux disease (GERD). This is a painful condition that if left undiagnosed and untreated can cause significant damage to the esophagus and gastrointestinal (GI) tract, Along these lines, constipation, whether due to diet, medications or simply an abnormally functioning GI tract can become a significant health concern.

He added that he has found migraine headaches to be a fairly common health concern for adults with autism.

I was curious as to what one should look for to determine if this kind of condition was developing in an adult with autism. He described symptoms of each concern: for seizures, one would notice "staring spells; unusual behavioral events potentially associated with the voiding of urine followed by the need to sleep; the eyes rolling upward into the head; herky-jerky (tonic-clonic) movements of the arms and legs when the person appears to be unconscious." With GERD, one would observe "a bending forward at the waist as if in pain; reluctance to eat associated with weight loss; putting fingers and other objects in mouth when this behavior hadn't been there previously; new onset loud vocalizations." Likewise, with constipation, you might notice the bending forward, and some pacing and maybe a change in eating habits. Head banging may indicate migraine headaches.

Dr. McDougle urged adult autistics to see their primary care doctors once a year as routine, but he remained concerned that this was one of the biggest challenges in autism adulthood. He advised that "it may be difficult to identify primary care doctors or medical specialists that care for adults with autism. They could begin by contacting local medical schools to see if they have developed such a clinic." In general, Dr. McDougle has found that the best place to start is "through word of mouth from other parents/caregivers that have been dealing with this challenge for a number of years. They are likely to know which medical providers are willing to see adults with autism, which seem to have a genuine interest in learning about and caring for adults with autism, and which are particularly skilled in working with this population. They might ask their pediatrician if they have had success referring their patients on for adult care and who they typically recommend."

Most frequently, the pediatricians remain the primary health provider throughout autistic adults' lives. Indeed, Nat is still with his pediatrician, although that is more because I've been reluctant to leave that wonderful nest, where all three of my baby birds have found the best of care for eighteen years. But I do know that it is time for Nat to move on. In our case, I will probably take him to my own PCP, who is a lovely man and very open-minded.

Another parent's quest for answers about autism catatonia

I talked to several parents at this time, because the parent network is the first stop in your climb up the autism learning curve. Liz from New Jersey has been dealing with her son Tyler's catatonia for several years.

Tyler's symptoms began eight years ago, when he was fourteen. Liz remembers that it seemed to start around Christmastime of that year. "Initially he was looking sad, losing affect, not getting that kind of excitement out of even Christmas that he usually has. He's a guy with few words but had always had a very nice affect. We have become pretty good at rationalizing and trying to explain behavior, and so attributed it to the [holiday] travel, a three hour time change, maybe a cold."

But a reduced reaction to Christmas was only the beginning for Tyler. "Even back in his home and school schedule we noticed he was slowing down," Liz said. "His after school routine had been to get off the bus, come in, take off his shoes, take off his backpack and put them in their assigned places. One day in January, ten to fifteen minutes after entering the house, I found him still at the front door, backpack on his shoulders, not having moved an inch. Almost frozen. This was a kid whom we had to constantly chase down when he was little, and here he was not even moving!" Tyler exhibited similar inexplicable stalling at shower time. Liz said, "I would get him up, get him in the shower and go check on another child. I'd find him having turned the shower off, not having reached for a towel. Standing there shivering."

Liz recalled more of the same unusual and frightening behavior at dinner: "It was time to start picking up plates. But he had not eaten. My fabulous eater had not even started touching his fork to his pasta. When I put a fork full of food to his mouth, he gobbled it down. As he lost weight over time, it became clear that he was hungry, but that he could not initiate eating. We had to feed him, like an infant, but without the crying. And he had even less to say than before." He lost thirty pounds, ultimately going from 135 to 105, between January and June. He was emaciated by the summer.

His doctor thought it was depression, and prescribed an increase in his tiny dose of SSRIs (Selective Serotonin Reuptake Inhibitor). But this only made him have incessant tics, and did nothing to improve his affect, language, appetite, or motor challenges. The SSRIs were tapered off and the tics stopped, but the deterioration continued. Tyler continued declining in numerous ways. "He looked like a ninety-year-old with Parkinson's," Liz said. "He would have trouble making it to the bathroom, so he'd have accidents literally standing in front of the toilet, because he couldn't get his pants down." And yet, there were signs that his cognitive functioning was still sharp. "One morning I let him sleep a little more. When I finally decided it was time to get him up, I pulled the covers back. There was this big white square in the middle of the bed sheets: he had cut out a perfect square where it had been wet." He had also managed to undress and put all of his soiled clothes in the hamper. "He was cognitively intact enough to know this was not a good thing. So he could not muster up enough motor planning to make it to the bathroom, but with the added impetus of embarrassment or discomfort, he had enough initiative and cognition to try to make it right." This extreme disparity signified a terrible problem to Liz. This was clearly another regression, different, but just as frightening and mystifying, as the one that occurred during his toddler years.

His doctor saw things differently. She felt that because he still showed these kinds of thoughtful, well-executed actions, he was not regressing. "Maybe it was semantics," Liz said, but both she and her husband Peter disagreed with the doctor. "Just as we were starting transition planning and thinking about the future in school IEPs, this was definitely regression. And how do you plan for the future when you aren't sure what tomorrow might be like?"

By that summer, Tyler had trouble with most kinds of movement, stopping and starting again, and then stopping, then at last mustering the energy somehow to complete an action. The stairs might take half an hour, and even getting in the car, for instance, was now an agonizing process. "He'd swing the car door, open-close-open-close, then finally shut. I started calling these 'body stutters,'" Liz said. "His arms would also move in these weird arm movements."

Peter and Liz talked to many experts in the autism world, and researched what they could online. At last one of their neurology specialists used the term "catatonia" on a Friday. By Monday, Liz had read what she could online, recognizing that like autism, this was another vague and terrifying diagnosis based on behavioral presentation that comes with no reliable test or solution. She and her doctors were also surprised to learn that, according to foremost autism research scientist Lorna Wing, catatonia occurs in "up to 17 percent of young adults with autism" (Wing, *British Journal of Psychology*, April 2000).

The initial literature that described catatonia in autism in its mild, moderate, and severe forms was enlightening, and in Tyler's case, the shoe fit. After some time in treatment and starting him on benzodiazepam, the doctor was excited to see the effects of the high dose lorazepam administered in her office, but Tyler's family knew that the effects were transient and that he would relapse into a largely immobile state shortly afterwards. His treatment at that point—a re-dosing every three hours—only yielded the same results: better affect and mobility for a half hour or an hour, followed by severely reduced movement again. It was clear that this "treatment" was only temporarily reducing symptoms and not addressing underlying issues; and even with times of improvement, Tyler's overall presentation deteriorated.

Despairing but undaunted, Liz continued to research symptoms and behaviors and called the doctor; convinced there might be a brain tumor involved. Highly skeptical of this possibility, Tyler's doctor nonetheless recognized that a full medical workup would be a good idea. The MRI scan showed nothing interesting, but the evaluating neurologist reported some interesting findings from a lumbar puncture, or spinal tap.

Testing revealed that Tyler had low levels of the measurable metabolites of the neurotransmitters dopamine and serotonin, as well as folate (Vitamin B9) in his spinal fluid. This explained some things—folate is critical to many processes, and dopamine is key to movement and visual perception. Serotonin is a well-known mood neurotransmitter, and all of these work in concert with each other and other key neurological processes.

While talking to me, I was struck by how learned and expert Liz sounded—how much she'd had to do by herself to help Tyler. Not only had she learned about these physiological dynamics down to the molecular level; she also had to observe Tyler acutely for even the most minute changes. Forget any possibility of normal living; the couple had to become scientists, psychiatrists, and neurologists and try to carry on even though their hearts were breaking.

But at last Liz and the doctors had begun to understand a little more about the symptoms. "I observed that his visual perception would really deteriorate throughout the day, and eventually I concluded that much of his anxiety was due to the fact that his depth perception was impaired. For example, in the evening, he'd get to a piece of furniture and stretch away from it as far as he could with a pinkie finger, keeping that as a reference to try to find something else to touch before he moved on. Open space was tricky, and he would hesitantly make transitions—from tile to wood, wood to carpet." Liz concluded that these unusual behaviors were likely due to the fact that he could not tell where things were compared to where his body was in space.

The introduction of high doses of folate brought significant recovery—enough that Tyler was moving better, less anxious, eating again—and the lorazepam was eventually discontinued. In the end it was the folate—a simple nutritive treatment—that did far more for him than the frequently used benzodiazepam. The form of folate was critical (5-MTHF or folinic acid), as researchers have learned that the folic acid present in our cereals, grains, and vitamin supplements can be hard for some individuals to break down, and as such get in the way of the body's needed form. Liz learned that most doctors and even nutritionists are not aware of this, or the fact that many of our medicines impair folate metabolism.

Still challenged by transitions, some body stutters, and a continued refusal to get on his beloved bike, Tyler began a new treatment. "He was given a dopamine medication called levodopa, frequently used in Parkinson's and the same drug that was used in the patients profiled in Oliver Sack's book and subsequent movie

Awakenings. This got him back on a bike and eventually running 5Ks with his dad," Liz said. "It was when we put him on the folate and added dopamine that Tyler returned to us."

Liz is a firm believer in looking under every rock, into every nook and cranny for answers, as well as doing a full workup (for Tyler, this meant blood, urine, EEG, MRI, CT scan, and spinal tap) to truly understand what might be going on in the body of an autistic patient suspected to have catatonia—or any other regression or significant change in behavior. For many of the affected families she has connected with since this has occurred, the route to a catatonia diagnosis was long, and even experts in the autism field are not aware of its penetration in this population.

Practitioners and caregivers need to be sure they are not merely ascribing changes or problems to "autistic behavior." This is a heartbreaking regression, and those left untreated continue to regress to a point where they might be tube-fed and bed-bound; that is not "just autism." "People with autism likely have an added vulnerability there because their neurotransmitter systems are already impaired," Liz said. "Just as with a tooth abscess or gastro intestinal concern, there are more health problems that persist in this population than in the mainstream; they often can't say what's going on and if they do, it is excused as part of the ASD." Therefore, one must delve deeply into the workings of their neurological connections and physiological conditions.

For Tyler, a reduced synthesis of dopamine and folate was likely key to the body's catatonic state. And yet, of course, this may not be true in other people, Liz cautioned, which is why specialists and parents must consider other possible causes, like GI or immunological issues, seizure activity, or even infections that may be undetected. There also seems to be some association between catatonia and a history of PANDAs (Pediatric Autoimmune Neuropsychiatric Disorders Associated with Streptococcal Infections). "So if there are new behaviors, [as we witnessed in Tyler], look for that infected tooth, sinus infection, or a GI problem. Ask if there can be exploration of an immunological component, a nutritional deficiency, or perhaps some sort of seizure component." Liz found that in working with Tyler's doctors, a picture—or a video—was worth a thousand words. "In comparing stories and examples of concerning or odd behaviors with other families we would get to that 'aha' moment of yes, this is what it is. I do think that catatonia is one of those disorders where some video examples would be helpful," Liz suggested. Parents and caregivers need online video examples of catatonia. But it might also be helpful to take videos of what the parent has observed to share with the medical team. One of the biggest challenges in diagnosis is trying to reduce the gap between how a typical parent would speak and how a typical doctor hears.

Unfortunately, syndromes like catatonia, or, as in Nat's case, a probable mood disorder, are not the first thing most doctors of adult autistics think of. In this way the medical profession is several steps behind the reality of autism adulthood. There needs to be a new kind of awareness: that adults with autism can develop further medical issues. If even close to 17 percent might have catatonia, this should be on doctors' radar, but it generally is not.

Therefore, Liz advised that the more parents know about the medical possibilities and their own child's case, and the more they can bring to the office visit, the more the doctor has to work with. She stressed the importance of connecting with other families and working toward a basic understanding of what might be occurring. "Researching symptoms helped—what I called moodiness, the doctors knew as 'emotional lability,' and what I called weird posturing was 'waxy flexibility' in their med school lingo. When I could use the terms that were in their heads, we made more progress."

Liz's most emphatic advice was that whatever the concern, a caregiver should observe his child, daily and over time. "Looking for patterns is very important." She stressed that eternal "must" for autism parents is, "If your instincts are that something's changed, something's different, keep pushing for answers. Things like catatonia and mood disorders are uncharted territory for us as families, but often for our doctors as well. My favorite doctors are not the ones who confidently tell us answers and send us on our way—it's the ones who sit and listen, and help to define the questions that still need to be answered, the unknowns that we explore together. The ones who don't give up."

A leading neurologist weighs in on the benefits of a multidisciplinary approach

After talking to Liz and some parent experts, I took my questions to one of my most trusted sources: Dr. Margaret Bauman, Boston University School of Medicine, Associate Professor of Anatomy and Neurobiology, and Child Neurologist at the Integrated Center for Child Development in Massachusetts. Dr. Bauman was the first doctor to definitively identify Nat's autism back in 1993, and we have since visited her for help with Nat during various stages of his life. When I asked Dr. Bauman for her thoughts on autism in adulthood and medical issues, she replied that my questions would be "tough to answer because of the fact that the recognition that ASD adults even exist, much less need health care, has only come to the top of the radar screen within the past few years. For many years, autism has been considered to be primarily pediatric, and many people still think of it that way."

This is why parents, caregivers, and self-advocates must come up with a plan of how to go about providing adequate healthcare to ASD individuals during adulthood.

"First of all," Dr. Bauman said, "everybody, including persons with disabilities, should be able to receive routine healthcare." There appears to be a new and increasing attention being paid to autistic adults at last, and the medical community is now becoming more aware of the fact that ASD adults can become ill with the same diseases as their non-autistic peers. What was once dismissed by professionals as "just being part of the autism"— meaning that there is nothing more you can do about presented symptoms other than treat them as a behavior problem, or quiet them down with medication—may now be taken more seriously. Dr. B. said, "I have a sixty-one-year-old, who is being cared for by her former sister-in-law and an advocate from one of the local Arcs, who finally got a pap smear and a mammogram for the first time." This represents an egregious failure in basic healthcare for autistic adults. Dr. Bauman fears that this execrable situation is more prevalent than not—and with males, too. "You have to wonder how many autistic adult males have prostate problems," she said. "So I'm not sure we need to be doing anything *special* here," she continued. "We should just be doing the regular things we do for ordinary people—but we're not."

Dr. Bauman talked mostly about what she saw as the heart of the problem in autism adult healthcare. First, there is the difficulty in finding adult practitioners familiar with the autism spectrum as a disorder. Equally challenging are the communication struggles that often accompany an autism spectrum disorder. Finally, my observations, along with others in the autism community, find a lower quality of life for many autistic adults in general once they leave school; this is associated with a lack of social and vocational stimulation, a sedentary lifestyle, meds that cause weight gain— any one or all of which may contribute to poorer physical and mental health than in the non-autistic population.

The National Institutes of Health have not yet definitively found this to be true, but there is a great deal of concern from what has been observed in the child autistic population:

> *It is unclear whether risk factors for obesity in ASD are the same or different from risk factors for children generally. However, obesity in ASD may be particularly problematic for a variety of reasons. First, core symptoms of ASD may relate to weight problems: for instance, children with ASD may lack social motivation to participate in family meals or in structured physical activities with other children, which might promote healthy weight. Likewise, families and therapists may be more likely to use food as a reward in children with ASD due to lack of social*

motivation. Many children with ASD also demonstrate selective eating as a restrictive/repetitive behavior pattern, and have been shown to have higher intake of low-nutrition, energy-dense food. The severity or type of a child's symptoms may also affect his or her ability to participate in physical activities that might mitigate weight gain. For instance, children with ASD who have a more depressive or withdrawn subtype may be less likely to participate in healthy physical activities or social eating patterns that protect children from unhealthy weight.

ASD comorbidities may also impact weight trajectories. For instance, poor sleep quality, which is common in ASD, may be both a cause and a consequence of unhealthy weight. Gastrointestinal (GI) disturbances, such as constipation, are also frequent in ASD and have been associated with poor dietary quality and obesity. Likewise, gross motor deficits, which are common in ASD, may prevent children from participating in age-appropriate physical activities that could mitigate weight gain. Safe and appropriate physical activity opportunities geared towards inclusion of children with ASD are often limited as well.

ASD treatments may also alter risk for OWT [overweight] and OBY [obesity]. The associations of common dietary treatments for children with ASD, such as gluten-free/casein-free diet, with weight status are unknown. Additionally, little is known about the effects of medication use on weight in children with ASD.

("Overweight and Obesity: Prevalence and Correlates in a Large Clinical Sample of Children with Autism Spectrum Disorder." Katharine E. Zuckerman, Alison P. Hill, Kimberly Guion, Lisa Voltolina, and Eric Fombonne, www.ncbi.nlm.nih.gov/pmc/articles/PMC4058357/)

According to Dr. Bauman, the medical profession in general is simply not prepared to take on the care of ASD adults. "Right now, many pediatricians are continuing to care for these patients because of lack of trained adult providers," Dr. Bauman said. "I'm a child neurologist—yes, I'm trained in adult neurology, that was part of my training—but I practice child neurology. Yet I'm seeing a bunch of adults because I don't know where else to send them." I have found this to be true for others in the autistic population, who remain indefinitely with pediatric dentists and primary care practitioners.

Given the complexity of the disorder and the limited availability of knowledgeable primary care and specialty providers to oversee the medical care of ASD adults, Dr. Bauman believes that, in the best case scenario, it would be important to create a clinical environment in which doctors from different disciplines could work together collaboratively, rather than working in silos. This seemed particularly wise to me: any particular specialist may be guilty of the "hammer-nail syndrome"—when all you have is a hammer, everything looks like a nail. Any one discipline may only be seeing through his or her own filter.

Dr. Bauman said, "Ideally you would have an in-house team located in a single site where providers from differing disciplines could confer with and learn from each other. It would be hoped that such 'teams' could be established in multiple sites, and that ASD adults could thus find needed expertise close to wherever they live." Dr. Bauman, for example, founded a clinic in Cambridge, Massachusetts about thirty-five years ago with other specialists, including a gastroenterologist (GI), psychiatrists, occupational therapists (OT), speech and language pathologists, an audiologist, neuropsychologists, physical therapists, social workers, and nurse practitioners. Given the heterogeneity of the autism spectrum, the multidisciplinary model makes the most sense, because "there isn't one discipline that can solve it all," she said. "You all learn from each other. I do believe that a lot of it is GI—but not all of it, of course." Dr. Timothy Buie, a leading gastroenterologist at the Massachusetts General Hospital, has taught Dr. Bauman a lot. For example, one of Dr. Bauman's patients was a twenty-four-year-old woman in distress. Her parents said, "We think she has headaches, because she says, 'head hurts.'" But Dr. Bauman's instinct and experience told her that this complaint was more likely about pain *somewhere,* not necessarily in the head. She recommended a gastrointestinal consult which yielded evidence of a gastrointestinal disorder which, when treated, resulted in no more "head hurts."

"What I learned about the presentation of gastrointestinal disorders in nonverbal patients I would never have known had it not been for my opportunities to interact with Dr. Buie. Similarly, I learned about sensory processing disorders because I was working with OTs there at the clinic. I learned from having those specialists around me and learned that when a patient presents with a behavior problem, the cause of the problem may not always be obvious."

Although Dr. Bauman believes that one's own primary care physician should have *some* resources to help them in the care and management of their autistic patients, the reality is that most PCPs may have limited experience and limited access to knowledgeable colleagues who can help them. She expressed great frustration with that fact. "Medical schools and training programs are going to have to do a better job in educating their students, interns, and fellows," she said.

These trainees need to be exposed to autistic children, adolescents, and adults during their clinical rotations, regardless of the specialty they are pursuing. In addition, those training in Masters or PhD programs working toward a research career in autism should also have opportunities to work with autistic patients, so that they have an appreciation of the variability and complexity of the disorder. I encourage the research assistants and graduate students working in my lab to spend some time in the clinic. I tell them, "Don't just spend time in the research lab, spend time in the clinic. Don't just read the book. Be with the patients."

Not all hospitals may have the comprehensive resources needed by the adult autism community. According to Dr. Bauman, hospital-based programs designed to serve the autism population can be expensive and, in many cases, not cost-effective. The patients are often time-intensive and complex, and reimbursement for time spent with these patients can be limited by the family's health insurance coverage. She said, "Each one of these autistic patients is different and their needs require an individualized approach, and that can be pricey." What's more, the staff may not be well-trained in how best to engage with autistic people. I've certainly found this to be true. I can't count how many times people have said, "Good boy!" to twenty-five-year-old Nat when he took off his shoes at their request. Or how often people talk about him right in front of him as if he isn't there, or does not have the ability to understand what is being said. However, with the advent of the increased availability of technology, including the iPad and other communication devices, it has become clear that a substantial proportion of the autistic population is not cognitively impaired, even if their expressive language and social interaction remain limited. Dr. Bauman learned this long ago, when a colleague's brother spoke for the first time at the age of fifty-five years. Up until then, he was completely nonverbal. "I think the fact that a lot of people have these communication devices has changed things. You can have someone who is very bright but nonverbal. I have become very cautious about what I say in front of my autistic patients, because I don't know who knows what. I assume competence until proven otherwise," she said.

So how does one go about finding the good professionals and helpful centers, and the specialists who have trained with patients and who know autism from that perspective? Dr. Bauman invested time, money, and energy pulling together her group in California. "When I first worked out in California," Dr. Bauman said, "finding the specialists I needed to help my patients was a real challenge. It took me eight years to find a gastroenterologist out there. It's not that there are no GIs out there, it's that a lot of them just don't 'get it.' I couldn't send families to someone who would blow them off. So I put a lot of these families on a plane to Boston. At least then they got care. Fortunately, I have since found three excellent gastroenterologists near the clinic in which I work and all three have become excellent and helpful colleagues." However, finding the right specialist for the right patient can still be a challenge. That is still the case, as we learned when we were trying to get in to see a catatonia specialist in New York City.

Dr. Bauman had higher goals, however. She wanted to build a team for her California families—but how? She decided that she would bring the talent out there. "I invited Dr. Buie out to California, and I took several gastroenterologists to lunch along with Dr. Buie. I wanted them to hear from the guru, and finally some of them got it. Now I have three!" Dr. Bauman has also since found an ear, nose, and throat specialist, an allergist, neuropsychologists, and two psychopharmacologists, and has access to excellent speech and language pathologists, occupational therapists, and physical therapists in the clinic in which she works. "You have to keep nibbling away at these problems. Even if it's not in the patient's backyard, a lot of people will travel," she said. "If the patient comes from a distance, however, we do what we can to network with colleagues near where the patient lives and attempt to find the needed high quality services close to the patient's home. Hopefully that would be the beginning of that patient's local team."

The key to a healthy autism adult life, though, is not only finding the right doctors, who understand the complexities of dealing with a person who has social-communication problems. Good health is also about creating an all-around healthy lifestyle, which comes from finding the right daytime activities, meaningful occupations, and social contacts. But Dr. Bauman has despaired over what she has found:

> At the present time, resources for ASD adults are very limited. In many cases, we haven't been able to be very creative in our day programs or with our vocational options. Some of my adult patients have reported being bored in their day programs. On the other hand, some families have arranged for meaningful employment and/or volunteer opportunities

for their young adults and many of these young adults have become very valuable employees in their respective job sites.

And so, it really may be that autistic adults may not necessarily have any more diseases or medical disorders than neurotypical people of similar age . . . I've seen patients with hypertension, diabetes, allergies, bladder and kidney infections, obesity, and large tonsils and adenoids. Many autistic adults can continue to have the same restrictive diets that they had as children, which can impact their overall health. Many are fairly sedentary and rarely exercise. If they're just sitting around, things can go south. They don't have a lot of activities, and even if they do, they might not be willing to get up and do anything. Similarly, the jobs that we provide for some of these folks may not be particularly inspiring.

Not that meaningful jobs and programs don't exist; they're just tricky to find—and sometimes they need to be created, as I've discussed in previous chapters. Dr. Bauman told me about one example of a terrific comprehensive day program out in California, where clients are trained for a career in film. "It is an organization called Exceptional Minds, started by a mom who has been connected to the movie industry. They have like thirty-five young autistic adults enrolled. Some of the clients there may even be nonverbal, but are taught how to use the technology, and eventually are able to work in film—like in *Avatar,* or *Hunger Games.* And they're paying jobs. They get their names in the credits."

In talking to Dr. Bauman, it became clear that whatever kind of service or specialist you're going to get, and whatever improvements in the system you're going to get, it will come from parents—on the personal level and on the advocacy level. To Dr. Bauman, the best resources are and have always been other parents. Parents have also always been behind the major changes in the disability community. Thus, it is the Arcs, the autism support centers, and the schools with special education parent advisory committees (SEPACs) of some kind that can be excellent sources for information on the best specialists, clinics, and professionals in the area. If you can find one parent to talk to and get some guidance, you're making progress. "Parents are going to have to drive this. To think the state is going to do this, or some university—no. If the parents don't do it, it's not going to happen, unfortunately."

Dr. Bauman is one of the chief pioneering autism researchers in the country, so she certainly believes in the importance of research, but not to the detriment of actual hands-on practice:

> *There's clinical and bench science research going on now, but how much of this research impacts those living with the disorder now is still elusive. Autism is now recognized as a heterogeneous disorder which can involve multiple organ systems including the brain, and which may have differing causes involving both environmental and genetic factors, resulting in differing neurobiologies and differing clinical presentations. All of this makes the search for effective treatments and interventions challenging.*

She talked to me a bit about mouse models and chimp studies. Such studies expand our body of useful knowledge, of course. We generally pursue animal studies with the idea that what we learn about biological mechanisms in these animals may one day be translated to help humans. However, occasionally, what we know about human disorders may in fact help animals, as illustrated by Dr. Bauman's chimp story: "My oldest daughter works at a large city zoo doing research. When I visited her, the staff in the research unit got to know me, and what I do. About three years ago I received an email from the staff indicating that they suspected that one of their chimps might have autism and asking me to provide a consultation. Observation of this animal found her to be demonstrating odd behaviors within the chimp group. I thought that this chimp might have a sensory processing disorder." Further observation by a sensory integration certified occupational therapist (OT) verified Dr. Bauman's suspicions. "We assembled a small group of experts including zoo staff, an anthropologist, neurologist, an OT, and a behavioral psychologist. They all concluded that the animal had a sensory processing disorder, and it was agreed to treat this animal much as we would treat a child with a similar disorder. A variety of sensory and motor activities were provided within the exhibit site and data was collected. It was theorized that chimps in the wild are constantly in cover, in the bushes, the trees, while in the zoo the animals are out in the open so they can be seen by the zoo patrons. We wondered whether this animal might be impacted by sensory overload. In addition to the 'therapy' provided, the staff created a covered site at one end of the enclosure. Data demonstrated substantial improvement in this animal's behavior as a result. I don't know if there is such a thing as an autistic chimp," Dr. Bauman said, "but ultimately the experience we were able to create had a positive impact on how the zoo handled its non-human primates. The observations resulting from this research project have since been reported at several scientific meetings and published in peer-reviewed journals."

Dr. Bauman and I have told the chimp story to lighten things up, but the experience does show that it is indeed possible to successfully diagnose and treat a nonverbal being—and please don't think I am at all comparing nonverbal humans to chimps. I am only talking about the principal of figuring out communication in challenging places. "Animal models are useful for figuring out mechanisms," she said. As is using what you have with an open mind to solve problems. We all need to gain inspiration somewhere. And in both cases, you just need the right specialists, in addition to having professionals who can infer a problem when the patient has trouble communicating verbally. Using augmentative forms of communication, like typing, pictures, and symbolic images, can be critically important.

We are still in the Stone Age in terms of autism adulthood and medical practices. Adults should not have to be going to children's hospitals their entire lives, nor should they be dismissed as "behavioral" when, instead, a GI exam might be called for. Therefore, self-advocates and caregivers must be proactive and be prepared to ask around and to move around until they find a doctor who seems to get autism. Being non-dismissive tops that list. Having a facility with alternative forms of communication is equally important. Furthermore, finding a practice that relies on experts from other areas of medicine is necessary so that you get the full picture of the medical complaint. Autism has its complexities, like any other disorder. In fact, so much can be learned about autism just by being with an autistic person, or by asking an autism person or caregiver what is wrong, what they may need—and then listening with an open mind. A behavior is not the end; it is merely an expression of a need or important problem. "All the research—we do need that, I get that, but for the folks that are here and now, they deserve better," Dr. Bauman said at the end of our interview.

Wandering, getting lost, and tracking

Some health issues are not about disease or diet or daily self-care. One of the most frightening items in the news about autism is the number of times our guys go missing. For us, all it took was that one horrible phone call from John, the summer Nat was twenty-five, and Ned and I became experts on tracking devices. It was around 4 p.m., long past the end of Nat's workday. John sounded like he'd been crying. He told me that he had only just located Nat.

They lived in a large apartment complex, nestled in several small streets of townhouses and rolling green parks. They had moved into an apartment there only days before, because John felt that it was safer and quieter, set back from busy streets. He needed off-street parking after our snow-laden winter of plows and buried cars on the Boston streets. And they needed a little more space.

Somehow, the bus company did not relay the new instructions about where to drop Nat after his day program. Danny waited at the apartment for Nat, and soon called John when Nat failed to show. John called the transportation company, only to be put on hold for twenty minutes. Hearts in their mouths, John and Danny searched for Nat and finally found him at the other side of the complex, headed toward the busy street.

He was safe. He had been trying to find his new apartment but there were so many of them and they all resembled each other. But Nat, John, Danny, and we were traumatized. And determined that this would never happen again.

But because we have all heard the horror stories of autistic people wandering, bolting, going missing, we needed to do more than swear at the bus company and swear that this would never happen again. We set about finding a way to protect Nat with a GPS tracking device. Here are some of the products we discovered:

Tracking Devices

- One friend of mine suggests a simple device you can get at Home Depot, a cheap alarm that is affixed to the door with double stick tape. You can take a set along for travel. It has an on/off switch. The alarm rings when the door opens.
- Eagle Eye is a security system that also does medical alerts: www.eagleeyesecurityinc.com
- Safety Net bracelet by Lojack: www.safetynetbylojack.com
- SmartSoles, a GPS tracking device in your shoe: www.gpssmartsole.com

- Have your house alarm set to go off every time the door opens.
- Autism Speaks' Autism Safety Project contains a lot of safety information: www.autismsafetyproject.org
- Project Lifesaver is a well-known and helpful organization, with a shop on the website: www.projectlifesaver.org
- Load the Family Locator app onto your cell phone, and everyone else's phone in your family: www.life360.com/family-locator/
- Ten lifesaving location devices for dementia patients: www.alzheimers.net
- These are ten wearable safety GPS devices for kids, some of which could be a solution for an adult: www.safewise.com/blog/10-wearable-safety-gps-devices-kids
- Pocketfinder's senior or child pocket locator is expensive, but worth looking into: www.pocketfinder.com

Tips for Autism Adulthood and Medical Care

- If you notice any new and unusual behavior, take note of what it is and when it began.
- Look for patterns in the behavior over time.
- Take videos of different behaviors.
- Don't wait for symptoms to worsen; see a doctor right away.
- Don't leave it all in the doctor's hands. Make suggestions of possible diagnoses and testing. Don't be afraid to be assertive; show and use what you know.

- Behaviors are only a manifestation: be sure the doctor looks into undetected infections, gastrointestinal problems, migraines, seizures, and allergies.
- If the diagnosis does not ring true, seek out a new doctor.
- If you don't have a good adult health practitioner for your autistic loved one, look for possible health providers at medical schools.

Resources (Note: some of these articles are a bit technical, but reading the abstract and skimming may help give you a fluency with the terms and concepts.)

- *Autism and Its Medical Management*, by Michael Chez, MD (Jessica Kingsley, 2009)
- "Catatonia in autism: implications across the lifespan," Dhossche, Wachtell, and Kakooza-Mwesige (*European Adolescent Child Psychology*, 2008)
- "Autism: is there a folate connection?" Leeming and Lucock (*Journal of Inherited Metabolic Disorders,* 2009)
- "Is there a connection between autism and bipolar disorder?" Jessica Hellings, MD, and Andrea Witwer (www.autismspeaks.org)
- "Bipolar disorder, schizophrenia, and other psychotic disorders in adults with childhood onset AD/HD and/or autism spectrum disorders," O. Stahlberg, H. Soderstrom, M. Rastam, and C. Gillberg (*Journal of Neural Transmission*, 2004)
- Organization for Autism Research's downloadable *Guide to Safety*: www.researchautism.org

- "Leaving the pediatrician: charting the medical transition of youth with autism," Marina Sarris (Interactive Autism Network at Kennedy-Krieger, www.ian.org, 2014)
- "Overweight and Obesity: Prevalence and Correlates in a Large Clinical Sample of Children with Autism Spectrum Disorder." Katharine E. Zuckerman, Alison P. Hill, Kimberly Guion, Lisa Voltolina, and Eric Fombonne (www.ncbi.nlm.nih.gov/pmc/articles/PMC4058357)
- "Accessible health care for autistic adults," Cynthia Kim (autismwomensnetwork.org/accessible-health-care-for-autistic-adults/)
- "Transition to adult health care for youth with autism spectrum disorders," Karen Kuhlthau and Marji Erickson Warfield (Association of University Centers on Disabilities, aucd.org)
- Exceptional Minds Studio (mentioned by Dr. Bauman as a terrific vocational program for people on the spectrum): www.exceptionalmindsstudio.org

CHAPTER TEN:

I CAN NEVER DIE, AND OTHER MYTHS

"Man plans, and God laughs."

—Sue from Massachusetts

THE OTHER DAY DURING A particularly difficult phase with Nat— months of extreme mood swings, periods of catatonic-like stillness followed by screeching laughter—I asked Ben, my youngest, if he was upset about "things these days." I did not need to be specific; Ben has an uncanny awareness of my own moods and the winding paths of my thoughts. He probably knew that I was probing gently at his long-healed post-traumatic stress from over a decade ago, when Nat's aggression was out of control. I guess I was expecting him to mutter something about how "yeah, he's fine, whatever," but that is not my Ben; he often surprises me with his responses.

"Nah. The thing I worry about, though," he said after a pause, "is how I am going to explain to him, make him understand when you are no longer coming back."

My heart flipped over. This was the strong, beautiful person he'd become. He'd always been sensitive and insightful, but as a little boy he had become so tangled in all of his emotions and observations. But those knots had fallen away like a thin necklace chain that suddenly unravels in your hands. I wanted to fold him into my arms and kiss him, but of course I stood where I was—he was seventeen at the time, and there was no way that was going to happen. So I chose my words carefully, to be sure they would soothe where my arms could not. "Oh, sweetheart," I said, "there's going to be a lot of other people in Nat's life—like now—who will be there for him, to explain about us, to take care of him like that. We're already making sure of that. But you know, when that time comes, you will have to make sure that *you* are OK. You'll have others to help you through it. You and Max will need to take care of each other."

"Yeah, I guess," he said, and the heavy moment lifted.

Reading between the lines of all these interviews, I realize that there's no magical answer to what to do for the future, particularly when we are no longer there. I've always thought that you have to find a person—a sibling, a paid caregiver, a family friend—who can do the basics of looking after your adult child later in life. Although we don't have our other children for the purpose of being their brother's keepers, they are indeed the natural choice for this later in life. That's the unsatisfactory truth. And yet, some families are more matter of fact about this possibility than I am. More than one autism friend of mine has said to me, on the question of siblings as future caregivers, "Yeah, well, that's what family is about."

What I do is every now and then, when it is germane to the conversation, I very softly let Max, and now Ben, know that they'll be overseeing Nat's living situation when we're gone. I also assure them that they won't need to do his day-to-day care but they will need to be checking in regularly to be sure he is being cared for properly.

Does this make me sad? Yes and no. I have to assume that I raised Max and Ben to be caring people, and that they won't take the easy way out with Nat, and not care what happens.

But it does make me sad thinking of the three of them making their way without my presence. But they don't need me that way, or at least, they won't by then. Not even Nat will, because he will be so used to living elsewhere and with others.

So what about the families who will have their autistic loved one stay with them, in their home? There has to be a way, there has to be something they can depend on when they're gone. What happens, generally? Does the state agency find them an opening in any old place? Is there always an opening, and if not, where do they go?

How can we prepare for the time when our autistic children can no longer live with us? When we die, if there's no house to shelter our child, no sibling to take him in, what happens?

A lifetime of planning leads to equanimity

Ann from Massachusetts has a son with autism in his forties. I talked to her on the phone about Paul's life and what she imagines the future will be like. She described his living situation as one that takes into account the long-term, because it is so simple to maintain;

> *Staff is there, but he doesn't need a one-on-one. He is in a program where he lives and works, a local program. We can go over there and visit and he can come home. During the day he has a job where he lives, separate from where he's living. He's part of the Clean Team. They clean up: do sweeping, laundry. They have a big commercial washing machine type of thing. Quite a bit of laundry to be done. They do the washing and the drying, and then they fold it. He likes doing that. Works every day—the job coach is shared with other people.*

Paul is quite independent, although challenged verbally. Yet like so many of the autistic adults I've come to know, he has had a lot of growth, perhaps because of so much continuity throughout the years. "More conversation now," said Ann. "He also understands sign language. He doesn't sign that much but he does understand it. Not every single word, but a lot. It enhances what he hears people say."

Paul has two other housemates, who are very different from him in personality and disability. Each one has his own bedroom. They live in what used to be a big furniture store. Paul works downstairs and he lives on the fourth floor. They have a big common room, with piano, tables, and couches. They congregate there, watch TV, plays cards, do puzzles. There's also a large living room, kitchen, and bath. Paul also goes out in the community, to the gym or a pool. "They're always going someplace," said Ann. "When I visit him, I say, 'Hi, how you doing,' and he'll say 'hi,' and give me a hug. He also comes home regularly and stays for a meal."

Paul's living setup has most of his support needs right there. On one side of the building—which was donated to the agency— are the director, social worker, nurse, and staff people whose offices are located there. It is a mixed use building: in addition to those directly associated with Paul's care, there is a dentist, senior residents, and a Democrat state representative even has an office there. Having other businesses there helps keep Paul and his roommates connected to the community. And I believe that the fact that the building was donated is a key to this living situation working out: this means fewer expenses for the families. If all they have to think about is food and perhaps a minimal rent to the agency, then they can be covered by SSI. Staffing still has to be paid for, and that, of course, is a large expense—far larger than housing—but still, this is one big piece that is solved.

The ratio for staffing is three clients to one or two caregivers. The staff rotates, like in a group home. But it does not have the feel of a group home. According to Ann: "It's like a family."

The big question in my mind was how Ann has planned for the future, when she is no longer there for him. "Well, I'm seventy-seven. The plans are for him to stay there as long as he can; hopefully his sister will watch out for him. None of us know how long we're going to live. The agency is so good that I really hope he can stay there. I've been with different agencies, and this particular one is good, because they have so much available."

I wanted to dig deeper with Ann; I wanted to find out how she keeps from being afraid of the future. "Everybody's different. He's forty-two. The agency has a senior program, a lovely home down the street. My dream has been when he's the age when he can go to that home . . . it will be good." Ann is confident that Paul will have the care he needs because he always has, for his entire adult life. They have been lucky with staff, so much so that Ann is very optimistic about her son getting good care even when she's gone.

"I have found the people who live with these people—they're very understanding and they do the best they can, physically, socially, they're there to help them." Ann's attitude was very like Diane's, who felt that someone eventually does step in. This calm perspective made me wonder: is it true that there are so many great caregivers out there? Or is it that there is a greater serenity to be found by the time you are a very old parent? Perhaps you just learn to have a certain degree of faith? But that can only be if you have been able to provide a satisfactory living situation for your loved one, all the way through. If your system has good "bones," a strong structure and layers of support, maybe that is the basis of a dependable future. Similar to Ann and Paul, we have a service provider overseeing Nat's shared living with John. They have monthly check-ins with John's supervisor, and John has vetted and trained Danny for extra help. The service provider has a nurse and psychologist on staff, and always he emergency back-up staff John can call—although, as illustrated by my story in the previous chapter, sometimes things move too quickly for one to stop and think who to call. We have to be prepared for sudden surprises and be able to think on our feet. When Nat was lost, getting dropped off at the wrong place, John rushed home to find him himself. He made a judgment call to handle it himself (and with Danny). He did not call the service provider, because he felt they were located too far away. I think he should have. Or perhaps he should have called the police. What's done is done, and we talked about this at length, and came up with a new understanding of how we would deal with such an event if it were to happen again. Open discussion is perhaps the hardest part of a caregiver-parent relationship, yet it is critical to make this effort.

And of course, Ned and I are firmly connected to Nat's life. I think about how, throughout Nat's life, I have tried to keep control of all the parts of his day. I have ways of checking in on him through the reports of others. His day program sends home a communication book, just like his teachers once did. I am in daily contact with his caregiver. I live close enough that I can visit at any point. But again, I wonder, who will do that when I'm gone? Will I eventually learn a way to let go, to let the others fill in the vacuum I will leave? This is so hard to contemplate as a fifty-two-year-old healthy, active mother. But maybe growing old means you are forced to let go and hope for the best.

There has to be careful planning, though. The habit of planning means you have created an infrastructure, a system of care and caregivers, resources, around your autistic loved one. This was confirmed by Ann: "Life goes on . . . as circumstances come up, if you are involved as we've been—we just kind of know the questions to ask and the people to ask." Ann and her husband have been on the Regional Advisory Board for the Department of Developmental Services for decades. No wonder they have some peace of mind. She has put her family on the system's radar screen. "You've got to be involved with the agencies and with the other parents," Ann said. "The hardest point is when they get older, turning twenty-two, and you've got to know what's going on."

Ann is not an autism sage—she doesn't claim to be, or need to be. She's an elderly parent who has learned over the years what questions to ask, how to assess her son's situation, and how to let go. Ann's achievements are not glamorous, not miraculous. They are specific to her son's needs, and they are not ideal by any stretch. But she believes he is safe, healthy, and happy. And so, because she can feel a certain peace of mind about her son, she is a role model for autism families. We have to remember that our goal is not perfection for our autistic loved ones, but nurturing a ground from which they can thrive and grow.

The future involves friends and family

Sue is trying to plan proactively for her autistic son, Ed. (Ed's living situation is detailed in Chapter Four.) The shared living home with a family (Kathy and her son) that he has known for half of his life recently came to an end. One of the integral staff members felt it was time to move on, pursue a different goal in his life. But the arrangement had been terrific for a very long time—fifteen years. "We would spell each other," Sue said. "Monday nights I would pick up both boys, and we'd walk in Worcester so Kathy had Monday nights off."

Ed's setup was a similar setup to our family's. We spell John by taking Nat on weekends. Frequently I help out with driving Nat places if John cannot manage it.

Sue had been hoping that Ed's shared living arrangement would work for him far into the future, but as she put it, "Man plans, and God laughs. The plan was that staff would live there with Kevin and Ed," Sue went on. "And in fact there was another young man living there, James." Kathy has known him for years. James worked with Ed Thursday nights, took him out into the community. They would walk at the mall, or on one of the tracks around town. Kevin and Ed enjoyed each other's company as well. They had complementary skills; Kevin liked to get his hands dirty ("Not keen on hygiene," Sue said), while Ed, on the other hand, showers, shaves, and brushes his teeth three times a day. Ed would work with Kevin in the yard for short periods of time.

Sue's description of the differences between Ed and his room-mate made me smile, because I remembered something John said about Nat recently, which moved me considerably: "Nat and I have the same personality. We both like to socialize, but we also need our space." As well as I know the two of them, this is true, and I'm so grateful that John thinks of Nat this way, as being just another guy with various needs and preferences. Of course John should feel this way—Nat *is* just another guy, after all—but how many of us really see someone like Nat as a psychological equal?

Being in a later stage of life than my family, Sue has to think about Ed's future without her. She and Kathy are in close contact, and so they are able to be very honest with each other about their future plans and needs. Kathy had been trying to fade out the high degree of support she herself offers. "Kathy has always been there as backup, but she's pulling away," Sue said. "Kathy would like to move away to Florida to retire, but this house has been in the family for generations. She wants to keep it for Kevin. She's built a bedroom in the cellar. Sometimes she'll be upstairs watching TV with them, but most times she's downstairs." Ed was really learning how to be more independent.

So when the living arrangement reached its end, Sue was disappointed, but not all that surprised. Like most other aspects of her life, Sue takes a pragmatic, rational view of the future. "It's never perfect. I don't lose sleep over it. That's about as much as a person can plan."

Although she is currently working on a new living arrangement for Ed, Sue has backup plans for him—Ed's sisters. "One is a board-certified behavioral analyst, so it's a natural support. She's always saying things like 'when's Ed's ISP?' Both of his sisters have always been this way. The other is a physical therapist." Sue believes that her daughters are also very nurturing. "I think it's a natural way of being for females. And for siblings, they feel they need to be responsible. One daughter has designated one room for Ed. Both have a commitment to him."

Ultimately, Sue has learned first and foremost that change happens—and often when you least expect it. She also wrote me later about autism and dealing with death. She told me that Ed has already had to deal with the death of several people in his life, so he may be able to handle that terrible time when she leaves him: "Three grandparents, two uncles, and an aunt. I explained that death meant someone's body was broken too badly to be fixed and that they went to sleep forever, and his response was, 'Gone and lost for ever,' a phrase he uses when something has been lost and can't be found. He showed various degrees of sadness and concern—mostly directed toward me as he comforted me. My feeling is that Ed has a similar concept of death as the general population—since if we are honest, most of us can't really fathom death."

Opting for more independence

Jane from Wisconsin is no ingénue when it comes to managing her son's housing and day programming. Her son Chris is forty. A single parent, no longer young, Jane has had to push tirelessly to secure the services Chris needs, especially with the future without her looming. When Jane and I first spoke, Chris had been living in what is called an Adult Family Home (AFH) in Wisconsin—a state-licensed and funded facility—with three other men who have been his housemates for fifteen years. But conditions in the AFH had deteriorated, and Jane was no longer satisfied.

Recently when Jane found a duplex that her daughter and her husband could live in with Chris, her feelings of hope for his future were restored. Her vision had been that they would occupy half of the house and Chris would live in the other half with roommates he has known for years. In her most recent email to me, Jane wrote that Chris was now living in the upstairs, but he was alone there—no staff person—with his sister and her husband in the downstairs. They now have an agency to support Chris, although Jane provides all backup support when staff cancel or do not show. "I think Chris will grow in many ways through this experience. And he will have the ability to choose what his day looks like."

Jane wrote, "We have staff from an agency providing support. It has not been easy and there has been lots of staff turnover. Overall, Chris is still happier living there than the adult family home."

Before she found the duplex, Jane and Chris had been unhappy with his living situation. "His adult foster home hired a new manager at his house, because last October Chris had a lot of behaviors, but that manager was awful. They wanted Chris out," Jane said. But Jane believed that Chris's challenging behaviors were simply reactions to the staff's animosity toward Chris.

How familiar that plaint is. The typical vicious cycle for our guys is that organizations often don't believe that they respond uniquely to each staff member. Some staff set Nat off, others have not. It is not fair to assume that someone has "behaviors" without looking at all the possibilities: one particular staff person or another may indeed be a catalyst, as I have found with Nat over the years.

Jane is optimistic that the duplex situation can work for Chris—as long as she is his director. It is a partnership, however, with Chris as the other main partner. "Chris *does* care about what happens to him. He shows it visibly through his behaviors. That's why I think moving him into a more independent lifestyle is working. He doesn't want you to help him. He shows pride that honestly I haven't seen before. I don't know where that's coming from. I'm getting a better idea of what he cares about. He does things for himself at work. When he's with me around the house, when he's with his sister, he'll cook and he'll bake, wash dishes, put things away, he'll find things. When he's here I have to stop myself from pulling something out of the fridge for him. He *wants* to do it."

Jane was not sure why Chris has become so active and invested in doing things for himself. "It might be because of the positive change at his house. He's very neat and orderly. The more positivity in his life, the happier he is, and the more he wants to do for himself. When he didn't have that, he suffered, he lacked self-esteem."

For Chris, language is also a barrier, but still he works in the community and goes to a day service. He has worked at one retailer for nearly two decades, which has not always been smooth, but his longevity there is remarkable. For autism families, there's often no stability in work, programs, staffing, or housing; it's constant change. And unfortunately, people with autism frequently have a difficult time tolerating instability and inconsistency. Jane said, "Chris can't understand why someone he likes would go away and he can't see them again."

Jane said that quality support staff means everything. "If you don't have that, what are the chances of success? Slim to none. But the core of the problem of finding the best support workers is salary, limited funding. No matter how experienced a parent or caregiver is, we always have to be prepared to go to the state agencies and complain. That never stops."

Jane said, "For me, the bottom line is safety and happiness/contentment. He might be more anxious than we'd like, but it is a new, stressful situation. That's the reality. His staff are good people, well-trained, and caring. That's another fact. His parents are highly involved, loving, but very intense. That's true, and it's okay." In the end, Jane has set Chris up for the indefinite future, but similar to most autism families, she can't be certain that his supports will continue to be there. Having his sister in the picture works for them, but of course that option is not for everyone and brings with it its own problems. Nevertheless, Jane has likely done all she can, and will have to hope for the best—like all of us.

A sibling firmly in charge

Susan from New York is in her early sixties. Her autistic sibling, Alan, is two years older. He was diagnosed with "everything, over the years," Susan said. Because he wasn't learning to speak, they thought he had aphasia; later that diagnosis was dropped. Then he was diagnosed as autistic, and that, too, was dropped. Then he was labeled mentally retarded (this is the outmoded term for intellectually delayed, but it was Alan's diagnosis at the time), and recently as autistic again. Like many of our loved ones on the spectrum, the IQ tests are not all that useful, and so no one could determine Alan's IQ—and Susan feels that they still don't really know.

Alan was in an institution by the age of eight. Prior to that, there were no programs or services available to him, other than a school in Manhattan. Once Alan turned eight, the school administration said they could no longer help him.

Susan remembers visiting him growing up. But eventually at some point she did her own thing, went to college, forgot about him, and didn't visit him for years and years. "My parents were going only every few months to see him," she said. "I think it was very painful. A lot of parents dropped their kids off at institutions and never came back."

Alan's place was Letchworth Village, the parent organization for Willowbrook, the institution that journalist Geraldo Rivera exposed in the 1970s for its atrocious treatments and living conditions. "Letchworth was beautiful, had an inspired mission at the beginning: everyone would work, they'd have a farm, animals. They were worked like slaves, though," said Susan. "They were not given jobs in the community." Over time, however, this changed and some did find employment out in the world.

The institution was twenty-five miles away from where Susan grew up, but psychologically and emotionally, the distance felt enormous. "My parents had a very difficult time," Susan said. "Once he went to the institution, they never mentioned him. No one knew they had a child like Alan. Having a child like Alan felt shameful back then, and no one talked about it. But it was the same with things like cancer. At that time, a million things were never discussed or mentioned. I stopped talking to my friends about him. It did a head trip on all of us."

Susan talked about the guilt and sadness people like her parents dealt with. I felt an old wound tear open as I listened to her. What she described is exactly how I had felt dropping Nat off at his first group home, at seventeen. Even though it was a nice enough place, in a cul-de-sac neighborhood with (mostly) caring staff, I went through a horrible period of pain over what I'd "done to Nat." Up until recently, in fact, I would still get a sinking feeling from dropping him off at the end of his weekend visits; a vague, poisonous depression would settle over me. Ned started going with me regularly to take Nat back, holding my hand on the way home and playing funny podcasts for me, just to help me get through the Sunday drop-off. Susan pointed out that her parents' guilt may not be too different from what parents like me feel at drop-off.

"People would say my parents were monsters," Susan said. "You become guilt-wracked seeing your child there, and having no control in what was done; if you brought clothes or if you brought him Christmas presents, it would be gone in a moment or circulated and given to other people. There was no way to have an impact on your own child's life. He became a ward of the state, no longer under the jurisdiction of my parents. He was like a convict."

And yet, Alan proved to everyone much later in life that society should never give up on people. Interventions work, even if they happen late in life. "Had he been growing up today, he would have learned to speak," Susan told me. She believes, as I do, that if someone has receptive language it is very possible that they can learn some kind of communication.

Most autism families and professionals would agree with this. I think of my autistic friend Dusya, who believes that schools ought to try typing or visuals with every single student who has autism—it is incumbent upon us, the majority, to do everything we can to elicit communication. No one should be cut off like Alan.

Susan began to forge a relationship with Alan when she started making a film about people in institutions. The film, *Without Apology*, became such an intense and cathartic project for Susan (and won some prestigious awards as well) that during its creation, she found herself able to come to terms with her brother as a real person, someone with whom she could connect. Susan said, "It was one of the first to tell such a full story of a sibling as a documentary (there was *Rain Man* up till then, but not much else), and it was the making of the film which allowed me to bridge the chasm—from alienated and uncomprehending to fullblown acceptance of my brother. I believe that telling one's story is often the path to 'liberation.'" For Susan, by the time the film was completed ten years later, there was no going back.

Alan had left the institution with no sense of initiative that he could do things. Susan said, "He did not even know, for instance, if he could take a tortilla chip out of a bowl without it being served to him. He had become so passive because of the training in the institution." After a few months, after letting him stop and start, she got him to understand he had power.

Susan began to become involved with Alan's program and medication in 1992, after her mother died and he'd been placed in a group home in the community. The adjustment was terribly difficult for Alan, Susan told me. "When a prisoner gets out of prison, they don't know how to adjust. He didn't sleep for a month. But then he got used to it, within three months." Eventually it became apparent to Susan that Alan's new routine was positive, and that his residence was a good one: a real house, in the suburbs, and much quieter than the institution had ever been.

"Faced with a wholly new system that demanded real participation, my father and I worked together. After his death in 2003, I chose to become legal guardian and advocated for my brother. A very different enterprise!"

"They fought me—being the sibling. The parent is listened to so much more than the sibling. Yet *I* was the legal guardian," Susan said. Although the situation is much better now, Susan still has to fight the system at times.

Much like older autism sibling Pam in Chapter Seven, Susan came to realize that as legal guardian she would need to know a lot more in order to fully understand her role. It turned out that she could indeed decree that Alan wasn't going to have any psychotropic medication, and as Alan's medical proxy, the administration and psychiatrist were supposed to respect Susan's wishes. But at that early stage, Susan didn't know her own power. She did not have that key information, which she emphasized was paramount to doing the guardianship right. "That is what has snafu-ed me at every turn. No one gave *me* a pamphlet," she said.

And so, like so many of us who advocate for our loved ones, Susan had to become tough and informed. This change in how Susan operated led her to become more aware of other aspects of Alan's care—she now handles her brother's money as well, for example. "I've sort of become a hard ass. I saw a suspicious line in his accounts and inquired about it—a one hundred dollar 'miscellaneous' item. Now I require the monthly statements." To educate herself, Susan got involved in Partners in Policy, which offered training in many aspects of special needs care, including the history of cognitive disability.

Unfortunately, Susan still feels frustration with the adult services system—yet another emotion I share with her, though we are decades apart in our experience as caregivers. "I learned that group homes are not all that different from the institutions. The guys are doing nothing wandering around, the television is on but no one's watching it." The institution had been like that too; the caregivers there exhibited a kind of "benign neglect," Susan found. "The group home has no 'home' in it. It's missing that quality. You're still at the mercy of the staff unless you can go every other day or so. I go once a month. Alan's music therapist goes every other week. She's also my eyes and ears," Susan said.

When Susan first took over as Alan's guardian in 2005, and even before that, she felt very alone, almost lost. There was no thought given to how things were for the siblings, how neglected they could feel. Susan was very glad when this changed, that there was so much more available now, and that siblings were getting some attention. Susan had joined a sibling support group as far back as the mid 1980s that was run out of the New York City Arc, which was helpful at the time. "One of the best things my parents did was introduce me to a sibling group. Mom got a flyer in the mail. That brought me into connection with these other siblings. They encouraged me to get back in touch with my brother. I'd lost touch with him for twenty years. I went to the institution myself many times." Like many other older adults caring for autistic loved ones, Susan has come to the conclusion that siblings do indeed most often become the caregivers once the parents are no longer there.

The sibling taking over for when I'm gone—that is precisely the answer I was hoping to avoid when I started this book. I wanted to find other strategies, other resources that would ease the burden of parents and siblings. I thought I could unearth some kind of buried treasure of respite and care for autistic family members. I wanted a magic bullet so that I could say it doesn't have to be you or the siblings.

But no, that secret cache of help isn't to be found behind a door at the DDS. The situation is far more complex than that. There are people who can help, but you must find them and cultivate them first. If you do it right, the sibling solution need not be the soul-suck many imagine it to be. As Don Meyer said, there is a full range of opportunities for the brothers and sisters to get involved, once they are ready. From visiting regularly, to guardianship as Susan did, or even to becoming the caregiver in a shared living situation, adult siblings can become a valuable and helpful force in the autistic family member's life. The key is to respect the sibling's full rights to his own life, dreams, and plans; to offer choices for involvement; and to offer support and information to ease that task.

The learning is by no means finished for Susan. She described the epiphany she had about Alan and music, while they were at a restaurant for his sixtieth birthday: "He loves eating out. He likes it so much that even after we'd sat around for a half hour without being served, he refused to get up and go. I had the embarrassing situation of calling the house and asking for their help. He's a smallish man but still a one-hundred-and-sixty-pound guy, and when he doesn't want to move, there's no moving him!" But Alan started acting out at this restaurant because they were taking a long time bringing them the food. "He was ready to eat," said Susan. "He started expressing his frustration loudly. I didn't know what to do. After all, this was kind of a nice place."

This scenario was very familiar to me: the anxiety Nat feels, the anxiety I react with, the frustration he must feel that no one understands what's bothering him, the mounting tension in the room. Over the years Nat has learned the routine and rhythm of eating in a restaurant. He loves to order for himself and to wait for the rest of us to finish before standing up. He is still learning how to talk more quietly to himself, an activity that he loves.

Music saved the day for Susan and Alan in the restaurant. "My cousin, a semi-professional musician, happened to be with us, and she had a recorder with her" Susan said. "She got her recorder, and played. He started moving to it. Then it hit me—what I should do is get some kind of music instruction or therapy. I found this wonderful woman who just loves Alan. She gives him a real one-on-one visit, steps in his shoes to see what to do each time, each week. Dancing, drawing together, playing instruments, listening to music on the iPad. With regular music he's been really progressing. He's coming out of himself. I can convey what I want from him. He can comprehend. He'll follow directions. It's just that the wiring is not the same as ours."

Susan ended our interview by saying, "I think that more and more, the siblings of these intellectually disabled and autistic adults will step in to help. There's a lot of reason for hope and optimism." I think that the fact that she ultimately feels this way is not only a testament to how things have changed for the better in our society, but also to herself, as a loving and caring sister.

Separation and letting go

How many times have I written about a new phase I've entered, where I'm letting go of Nat to some degree? It kind of makes me laugh cynically, because of course I don't hold onto that progress. Maybe none of us do. I used to say that the emotional cycles of autism caregiving come and go and come back again, and that is still true.

Now that Nat is in his mid-twenties, where I am is new(ish) for me. He has a fairly settled life as an adult at this point. He lives happily in his apartment during the week, works at the supermarket, and does part-time day habilitation weekdays as well.

Even though it would be easy for me to hear about how Nat's days at his program go, the truth is I only find out the bad things during the week. As vigilant as I am, I don't check in as much as I should. The way it works is I'll get a call from the day program about how depressed he seems, or how he threw something. Just like all the years of his youth, the aggression comes "out of the blue"—no one has a sense of precedent, and definitely not an antecedent. No one takes that kind of data in adulthood. There is a letting go in all parts of his life in the name of adulthood. He's an adult with moods and bad days like any of us, and so to some extent, we can't know and we only intervene when things get violent.

My own independence from Nat is going to be a lifelong process.

State House story

In February of 2015, a friend called and asked me if I had any suggestions for speakers on Autism Awareness and Acceptance Day at the State House.

I had been a speaker on Autism Awareness Day back in 2006 but the most exciting Autism Awareness Day I'd ever attended by far had been the very first, when one of the guest speakers had stood up at the podium with his mom, a longtime activist. The young man was in his early twenties, and had a developmental disability. I don't remember if he actually spoke, but I do remember his stage presence, his proud posture, his adult demeanor, and I remember thinking, "Wow. How does that even happen?" I was, of course, wondering what Nat would be like when he was that age. There was a small, smoldering sadness behind my eyes, which back then was so familiar. In those days, I was always looking at Nat with so much worry about who he would become. He was a young teen then, and had accomplished so much with his life: he was on team sports, had had a bar mitzvah, was a comfortable traveler, an excellent student. But I was focused on grown-up Nat, unknown Nat. Out-in-the-world Nat. And most of the time when I thought of him, it was with the sweeping, protective, despairing love of Mrs. Jumbo, Dumbo's mom.

But I put that pain aside and went back into my life at the time, raising my boys, writing books, and attending and speaking at events like AFAM. When I got the call from one of the organizers that winter day, I thought about one or two young men I knew who could possibly speak about their adult lives for Autism Awareness Day 2015.

As we were talking, though, the organizer made it clear that they were looking for a speaker who had fairly severe autism—someone who represented the end of the spectrum that is rarely written or talked about. I thought of Nat right away, and volunteered him as a speaker, with John to round it out. Why couldn't Nat do it, after all? He could answer questions as long as they were shaped around specific information. And he could type his answers. He could construct a speech about shared living, which was one of the topics scheduled for that day.

Ned, of course, was a little skeptical when I told him. This was our old familiar pattern of my big floaty dreams being met with Ned's rock solid sense of reality. "It might be too much for him," Ned said. "I don't know if he'll be able to focus."

I would not hear this. "He'll love it. He's great with crowds. He'll practice the speech. It will be just like his bar mitzvah."

Ned would not give me the satisfaction of agreeing and getting excited about it with me. But that was all right. It was going to happen. And I knew that whatever "it" turned out to be would be okay. That great hall at the State House was going to be filled with friends, autism families, advocates, and legislators who knew about Nat or, if not, would just love him when they saw him.

I'd come a long way since those days when he was fifteen. More importantly, so had Nat. The process went just the way I thought it would—a tribute to my deep familiarity with Nat's abilities and his favorite pastimes. Typing answers to questions was something he felt strongly about, after all. I told him: "Some friends have asked if you want to talk about your life with John, for a special day in the spring, in April."

He said "Yes" right away. So I told him about how he would create a speech, and that by reading it to the crowd he would be helping others understand how to live in an apartment and have a job, like he did.

He eagerly sat with me, laptop open, eyes strained as if to catch the words I spoke. I asked him questions like, "Nat, where do you live?" And he would answer.

"Okay, type that," I'd say. If he got lost I would repeat his own words, and restart him. After about a half hour, we had seventy-three words about Nat's experiences with shared living. Here is the speech:

> *Thank You*
>> *Living at Kelton Street. by Nat Batchelder*
>> *Brought Bag up stars to apartment at kelton street*
>> *At Kelton Street I eat Lunch go to bed sope and shawor, get ready pajamas go to bed*
>> *Jon coms, says get up*
>> *Brush teeth*
>> *Go to ASA Do meals on wheels*
>> *Back to Kelton Street. movies with jon. Put plates in dishwasher. set table. put datergent Lindre in drire*
>> *Feel happy*
>> *love nat*

Better than most speeches one hears at the State House, don't you think?

The night before Nat's speech, I didn't sleep very well. I knew I didn't have any reason to be nervous, exactly. I guess it was just that I didn't want Nat to feel uncomfortable once he got up there and actually faced all those people. I kept trying to tell myself he would be fine, that he doesn't get worked up when he's scared or when places are noisy and crowded. The episodes he has had with acting out are always about a sudden change in routine combined with his confusion and inability to formulate questions. And without being able to question us, he becomes choked with frustration.

I rushed through getting dressed, changed my outfit many times, although I don't know why—after all, this was not my show, but old egos die hard. I found Ned there and my old buddy Jeff, too, who had come there for Nat. A steady stream of fellow autism parents and professionals from over the years came up to me and wished me luck. Some had brought their children—budding self-advocates. Some were giving their own speeches. It was a warm sea of friends, buoying each other up, as we always did.

Nat was not there, but of course I kept scanning for him. I looked at my phone and there was a text from John: "It's on Beacon Street, right?"

Ahhh! John! That same old laid-back, huge self-confidence. Was he seriously not even inside the State House yet? I was back to my bouncy nervous state.

Five minutes later Nat strode in, glowing in his dove gray suit and silver striped tie. I gave him a kiss and gave John a hug. Nat was wired, but in a good way. I dug a pile of papers out of my bag: I had copied Nat's speech to hand out to everyone so they could follow along. I guess I was obsessing about people not being able to hear him or understand his quick way of reading. My hands were shaking and I suddenly felt shy going up to people with my son's speech. So a friend came to my rescue and had her sons take over distributing them for me. I found Nat a seat in the front row, and we all settled in.

The governor was ahead of Nat in the order of the program, and he gave a warm, sometimes funny speech, telling us stories about his experiences with autism families.

Then it was Nat's turn. He seized hold of the podium and began almost immediately.

You could not hear a thing, though his lips were moving correctly over his written page. One of the speakers—an autism mom who had created her own day program and residence—got up to push the mic closer to Nat. I still could not hear him. Dammit, I thought. Here I go. "Louder!" I shouted.

Nat shouted into the mic for one phrase, then went right back to his whisper. And I sat there feeling like an idiot because I had stepped in like a pushy stage mom and interfered with this young man's speech.

But really, what would anyone expect from me? That's the kind of mother I am, and I am the kind of mother Nat needs.

In the end, I don't believe Nat cared. He finished his speech, in his softest, quietest voice. But it was the voice of one of our guys, and it so roared like thunder within those marble halls.

Resources for Dealing with the Death of a Loved One, and for Letting Go

Books and Articles

- To help someone with autism deal with the death of a loved one, take a look at *Autism and Loss*, by Rachel Forrester-Jones and Sarah Broadhurst (Jessica Kingsley Publishers, 2007).
- Check out the following article on talking about death with an autistic person: www.ukautism.org/pdf/compass/understandingdeath.pdf
- Author Liane Kupferberg Carter is a fellow autism mom and friend who has a great blog post about helping her

autistic son deal with the grief over the death of a pet: www.autismafter16.com/article/10-15-2013/saying-goodbye
- "Navigating Grief and Loss as an Autistic Adult," Lynn Soraya (*Psychology Today*, December 2014)

Online

- Take a look at Gray Miller's "Being Autistic and Dealing with Death": autism.lovetoknow.com/Being_Autistic_and_Dealing_with_Death
- Although aimed at the younger autism population, many of the points apply: www.expertbeacon.com/helping-kids-autism-spectrum-disorder-navigate-bereavement
- This is aimed at children, but is still helpful advice: www.blog.stageslearning.com/blog/understanding-death
- On coping with death: www.carautismroadmap.org/coping-with-death/
- This document from Emarc, a Massachusetts area arc, is a great planning resource, so that future caregivers will know what your loved one's needs are: www.ndss.org/PageFiles/3022/footprints_for_the_future.pdf
- The website Pathfinders for Autism has some tips on discussing death with an autistic person: www.pathfindersforautism.org
- Autism Speaks has a section on their website with books and ideas for talking about death and bereavement with an autistic loved one: www.autismspeaks.org/family-services/resource-library/bereavement-and-grief-resources

EPILOGUE

W HAT IS THE FINAL WORD for caregivers, loved ones, and self-advocates dealing with autism in adulthood? Legwork. Advocacy. Vigilance. Lists. Keep making lists of what you need to learn, whom you need to contact, resources you have found. Along with "lists" comes "ask." Ask people what you don't understand. Buy them a cup of coffee for an hour of their time. Other parents and people in the field are mostly very happy to help the next generation coming up.

I'm sorry, I wish I could tell you otherwise, but there is no magic bullet other than hard work, pushing, staying on top of the offerings, strategies, resources, and laws that will make our guys' lives worth living. And the way you start is by talking to others.

So take a deep breath and dive in.

Now . . . let's take a new look at my death scene from chapter one:

And so, here I am—eighty years old? No, make that ninety-two. Falling into my last sleep.

Ben, my youngest, his dark brows lowered in his own sadness, notices Nat's distress. He has had a lifetime of reading Nat and fixing things so that Nat can have his routines. Whether out of concern or damage control, Ben learned long ago what to do. "It's okay, Nat," he says, moving closer to him.

Max looks around at them and murmurs, "Hey Nat." He shuffles over. His eyes are bright blue, now crinkled at the corners—just like Ned's were.

Ben and Max bookend their brother, who is still hunched, making little humming sounds around his thumb. They are blurry to me. My heart is squeezing this one last time as I feel their presence, my three boys.

Consciousness fades in and out.

The room is a heavy quiet, except for Nat, whose anxiety almost parts the air with its energy. "Mommy will wake up," he says again. And then, an arm drops around Nat's shoulders. John's smiling dark face is creased—he's old, too, his tightly curled hair is peppered with wiry gray. He may not be Nat's caregiver anymore, but he is here with him, forever the older brother. "Nat, it's okay. She needs to sleep. Okay? Remember, we talked about Mommy's long nap?"

Nat is listening, but he is watching me. He takes his hands out of his mouth. "No long nap." Every now and then, Nat still sucks his thumb. Seems like a very silly thing to worry about now—why did it matter so much?

He brings his clasped hands to his face again, drawing on his thumb. Faintly I hear the chirping, the oldest sound from motherhood.

"Okay? We have to let Mommy sleep a lot," John says, his voice uncharacteristically soft. "Okay, Nat?" He knows from over the years that you have to say "okay" a lot and you have to look Nat in the eye and make sure he says "okay" back. Nat has to have the okay-response in order to move on to the next thing.

"Okay," he says through his thumb. His voice sounds wet, nasal. "Okay."

"Come on, Buddy," says John, pulling him back, turning him, gently. "Let's give Mommy a kiss."

Nat's face as an older man is rough, his lips are dry. I feel them brush my cheek, old leaves blowing across the November sky. Nat will always give you a kiss if asked.

John says, "Let's go get a treat."

"Yes."

* * *

And so the only thing I can do is plan, and find people like John for him. Have the loose ends tied up as much as possible. Make sure Max and Ben are connected to him—and a support group.

Until my long nap comes, I can only be Nat's mom. Oh, thank God. Great to get some perspective, right?

I can continue to set up his social life, his Special Olympics training, his holiday celebrations. I will keep spying on him at work, and checking in obsessively with his caregiver. The eternal questions, "Is he okay? Is he happy?" are going to be on my mind. He feels it, right? I hope he feels it. I hope he can feel it even when I'm not there physically anymore.

Now that I've finally expressed these awful thoughts, I *have* to see him. Friday can't come soon enough. He visits us every weekend. I will go and take him out for a treat. Breathe him in, his young warm face pressed against mine. We can go anywhere, do anything. Now, while we're still here on earth, the sky's the limit—not autism. All we can do—any of us—is love each other, for as long as we're alive. And go get as many treats as possible.

RESOURCES

WEBSITES

General Autism Information: The Biggies

- Arc of the US: www.thearc.org/
- Autism Society of America: www.autism-society.org/
- Autism Science Foundation: autismsciencefoundation.org
- Autism Self Advocacy Network: autisticadvocacy.org/
- Autism Speaks: www.autismspeaks.org
- Organization for Autism Research: www.researchautism.org

Inspirational

- *Diary of a Mom,* Jess Wilson's blog: adiaryofamom.com/
- *Making a Difference:* www.kerrymagro.com/philanthropy/
- *Susan's Blog,* www.susansenator.com
- *Invisible Strings:* theinvisiblestrings.com

- *Carly's Voice:* www.carlysvoice.com
- *Thinking Person's Guide to Autism:* www.thinkingautismguide.com
- *Kim Stagliano:* www.kimstagliano.com
- *ThAutcast:* www.thautcast.com

Work and Education

- Do2Learn: www.do2learn.com/JobTIPS
- Pivotal Response Therapy (PRT): www.autismprthelp.com
- AbleLink Technologies: www.ablelinktech.com/index.php?
- Attainment company offers an abundance of assistive technology: www.attainmentcompany.com/product-categories/app-central
- Fraser: www.fraser.org/Resources/Products/QuickCues.aspx
- Exceptional Minds Studio: www.exceptionalmindsstudio.org
- Ocali: www.ocali.org/project/tg_employment
- Arthur and Friends Hydroponics: www.arthurandfriends.org
- Rising Tide Car Wash: www.risingtidecarwash.com
- The Teaching Hotel, Arc of Indiana website: www.erskinegreen-institute.org/
- Roses for Autism: www.rosesforautism.com
- Lee and Marie's Cakery: www.leeandmaries.com
- Stuttering King Bakery: www.stutteringkingbakery.com
- Autism Speaks: www.autismspeaks.org/family-services/tool-kits/employment
- Agricultural Communities for Adults with Autism: http://ac-aa.org
- Department of Labor's Workforce Recruitment Program: www.dol.gov/odep/wrp
- Autistic Self-Advocacy Network: www.autisticadvocacy.org/projects/books/navigating-college
- College Steps: www.collegesteps.org
- Taft College: www.taftcollege.edu
- Arc of the US's Autism Now initiative: www.autismnow.org/on-the-job

- National Adult Day Services Association: www.nadsa.org
- College Internship Program (CIP): www.cipworldwide.org

Housing Help

- Autism Housing Pathways: www.autismhousingpathways.net
- A Place Called Home: www.allenshea.com/CIRCL/documents/ SingleHouseSLS.pdf
- Juniper Hill Farms: www.juniperhillfarms.org
- "Twenty-Two at Twenty: A Nontraditional Transition Story", Cheryl Ryan Chan: www.slideshare.net/cherylryanchan
- First Place: www.firstplaceaz.org
- 3L Place: www.3lplace.org/living.html
- Camphill Association of North America: www.camphill.org
- Adult Foster Care: www.medicaid.gov/federal-policy-guidance/ downloads/faq-12-27-13-fmap-foster-care-chip.pdf
- Advocates, Inc.: www.advocates.org

Benefits, Staffing, Caregivers

- Medicaid: www.medicaidwaiver.org/
- Disability Benefits 101 in California: www.ca.db101.org/ca/situations/youthanddisability/planning/program2d.htm
- www.care.com
- Rewarding Work: www.rewardingwork.org
- Craigslist: www.craigslist.com

Medical, Emotional, and Safety Resources

- AASPIRE: www.autismandhealth.org
- Although aimed at the younger autism population, many of the points apply: expertbeacon.com/ helping-kids-autism-spectrum-disorder-navigate-bereavement

- This is aimed at children, but is still helpful advice: www.blog. stageslearning.com/blog/understanding-death
- This document from Emarc, a Massachusetts area Arc, is a great planning resource, so that future caregivers will know what your loved one's needs are: ndss.org/PageFiles/3022/footprints_ for_the_future.pdf
- The website Pathfinders for Autism has some tips on discussing death with an autistic person: www.pathfindersforautism.org
- Autism Speaks has a section on their website with books and ideas for talking about death and bereavement with an autistic loved one: www.autismspeaks.org/family-services/ resource-library/bereavement-and-grief-resources
- Eagle Eye Security: www.eagleeyesecurityinc.com
- Lojack: www.safetynetbylojack.com
- SmartSoles: www.gpssmartsole.com
- Autism Speaks's Autism Safety Project: www.autismsafetyproject.org
- Project Lifesaver: www.projectlifesaver.org
- Family Locator: www.life360.com/family-locator/
- Ten Lifesaving Location Devices for Dementia Patients: www. alzheimers.net
- Ten Wearable Safety GPS Devices for Kids: www.safewise.com/ blog/10-wearable-safety-gps-devices-kids
- Pocketfinder: www.pocketfinder.com
- Home Depot's door alarms: www.homedepot.com

Social Skill Resouces

- ACT Programs from the Governor's Council of Minnesota: www.selfadvocacy.org/programs/workskills.htm
- Developmental, Individual Difference, Relationship-based (DIR): www.icdl.com/DIR
- Healthy Transitions: Moving from Pediatric to Adult Health Care, and New York State Institute for Health Transition Training: www.healthytransitionsny.org.

- "Speak it!": chrome.google.com/webstore/detail/speakit/pgeolalilifpodheeocdmbhehgnkkbak
- Between the Lines Advanced (for Adults): www.itunes.apple.com/us/app/between-the-lines-advanced-hd/id574685561?ls=1&mt=8
- Job interview coaching software: www.jobinterviewtraining.net
- The Autism Research Institute: www.autism.com/news_agi_ebulletin
- A sexual health toolkit: http://www.bcchildrens.ca/our-services/support-services/transition-to-adult-care/youth-toolkit/sexual-health
- TASH (originally stood for The Association for Persons with Severe Handicaps) Conferences: www.tash.org
- iAssist Communicator: www.iassistcompany.com
- Organization for Autism Research, www.ow.ly/HMkaN
- Special Olympics, www.specialolympics.org

Sibling Help

- Sibling Leadership Network: www.siblingleadership.org
- Sibteen Facebook: www.facebook.com/groups/SibTeen/
- Organization for Autism Research's Sibling Support Initiative: www.researchautism.org/family/familysupport/SiblingSupportInitiative.asp

BOOKS

Inspirational and Thought-Provoking

- Jennifer Boylan, *She's Not There,* (Broadway Books, 2013*).*
- Arthur Fleischmann, *Carly's Voice: Breaking Through Autism* (Simon and Schuster, 2012).
- Robison, John Elder *Look Me in the Eye (*Three Rivers Press, 2008).
- John Elder Robison, *Raising Cubby* (Crown, 2013).

- Susan Senator, *Making Peace With Autism: One Family's Story of Struggle, Discovery, and Unexpected Gifts* (Shambhala, 2006).
- Steve Silberman, *Neurotribes: The Legacy of Autism and the Future of Neurodiversity* (Penguin, 2015).
- Stephen Shore, *Beyond the Wall: Personal Experiences with Autism and Asperger's Syndrome* (Autism Asperger Publishing Company, 2003).
- Laura Shumaker, *A Regular Guy: Growing Up With Autism* (Landscape, 2008).
- Chantal Sicile-Kira, *A Full Life With Autism: From Learning to Forming Relationships* (St. Martin's, 2012).
- Ron Suskind, *Life, Animated: A Story of Heroes, Sidekicks, and Autism,* (Kingsfield, 2014).
- Daniel Tammet, *Born on a Blue Day* (Free Press, 2007).

Social Skills, Sexuality, and Finance Guides

- Melissa Dubie and Judy Endow, *Learning the Hidden Curriculum* (Autism Asperger Publishing Company, 2012).
- Karri Dunn Buron, *A 5 Is Against the Law! Social Boundaries Straight Up! An Honest Guide for Teens and Young Adults* (Autism Asperger Publishing Company, 2007).
- Rachel Forrester-Jones and Sarah Broadhurst, *Autism and Loss,* Jessica Kingsley Publishers, 2007).
- Valerie L. Gaus, PhD, *Living Well on the Spectrum: How to Use Your Strengths to Meet the Challenges of Asperger's Syndrome/ High-Functioning Autism* (Guilford Press, 2007).
- Temple Grandin and Sean Barron, *The Unwritten Rules of Social Relationships: Decoding Mysteries Through the Perspectives of Autism* (Future Horizons, 2005).
- Temple Grandin and Kate Duffy, *Developing Talents: Advice and Strategies for People on the Autism Spectrum.* (Autism Asperger Publishing Company, 2008).

- Lynn Kern Koegel and Claire S. LaZebnik, *Growing Up on the Spectrum: A Guide to Life, Love, and Learning for Teens and young Adults with Autism and Asperger's* (Penguin, 2009).
- John Miller, *Decoding Dating: A Guide to the Unwritten Social Rules of Dating for Men with Asperger Syndrome (Autism Spectrum Disorder)* (Jessica Kingsley, 2014).
- Haley Moss, *A Freshman Survival Guide For College Students with Autism Spectrum Disorders* (Jessica Kingsley, 2014).
- Valerie Paradiz, *The Integrated Self-Advocacy ISA™ Curriculum: A Program for Emerging Self-Advocates with Autism Spectrum and Other Conditions.* (Autism Asperger Publishing Company, 2009).
- Kate E. Reynolds and Jonathon Powell, *Sexuality and Safety with Tom and Ellie book series* (Jessica Kingsley, 2014).
- Susan Senator, *Autism Mom's Survival Guide (For Dads, Too!)* (Shambhala, 2010).
- Brenda Smith Myles, Judy Endow, and Malcolm Mayfield, *The Hidden Curriculum of Getting and Keeping a Job: Navigating the Social Landscape of Employment: A Guide for Individuals With Autism Spectrum and Other Social-Cognitive Challenges.* (Autism Asperger Publishing Company, 2012).
- Lynn Soraya, *Living Independently on the Autism Spectrum*: *What You Need to Know to Move into a Place of Your Own, Succeed at Work, Start a Relationship, Stay Safe, and Enjoy Life as an Adult on the Autism Spectrum* (Adams Media, 2013).
- Zosia Zaks, *Life and Love: Positive Strategies for Autistic People* (Autism Asperger Publishing Company, 2006).

Safety and Medical Concerns

- Michael Chez, MD, *Autism and its Medical Management* (Jessica Kingsley, 2009).
- Melissa Dubie, *Intimate Relationships and Sexual Health: A Curriculum for Teaching Adolescents/Adults with High-Functioning*

Autism Spectrum Disorders and Other Social Challenges (Autism Asperger Publishing Company, 2011).
- John S. Roland, *Families, Illness and Disability: an Integrative Treatment Model* (Basic Books, 1994).

Sibling Help

- Paul Karasik and Judy Karasik, *The Ride Together* (Washington Square Press, 2004).
- Elaine Mazlish and Adele Faber, *How to Talk so Kids Will Listen and Listen so Kids Will Talk* (Scribner, 2012).
- Mary McHugh, *Special Siblings: Growing Up With Someone With a Disability* (Brookes Publishing, 2002).
- Don Meyer and Emily Hoe, eds., *Sibling Survival Guide* (Woodbine House, 2014).
- Jeanne Safer, *The Normal One* (Delta, 2003).
- Bob Smith, *Hamlet's Dresser (Scribner, 2003).*
- Kate Strohm, *Being the Other One* (Shambhala, 2005).

ARTICLES

Social and Financial Guides

- Brent Betit and Dorie Clark, "How to Work with Someone with Autism," article in *MarketWatch* www.marketwatch.com/story/how-to-work-with-someone-with-autism-2015-02-11
- Naomi Karp, "Managing someone else's money," www.consumerfinance.gov/blog/managing-someone-elses-money
- Lynn Soraya, "Navigating grief and loss as an autistic adult," (*Psychology Today,* December 2014)
- UK Autism "Understanding Death," www.ukautism.org/pdf/compass/understandingdeath.pdf

Medical and Emotional Crisis Help

- Autism Love To Know: autism.lovetoknow.com/Being_Autistic_and_Dealing_with_Death
- Liane Kupferberg Carter, "Saying Goodbye," www.autis-mafter16.com/article/10-15-2013/saying-goodbye
- Coping with Death: www.carautismroadmap.org/coping-with-death
- Dirk M. Dhossche, "Decalogue of Catatonia in Autism Spectrum Disorders" (*Frontiers in Psychiatry,* 2014).
- Dhossche, Dirk. M, Wachtell, and Kakooza-Mwesige "Catatonia in autism: implications across the lifespan," (European Adolescent Child Psychology, 2008).
- Dhossche, Wachtell, and Wilson, "Catatonia in childhood and adolescence: implications for the DSM-5" *(Primary Psychiatry,* 2010).
- Jessica Hellings, MD and Andrea Witwer, "Is there a connection between autism and bipolar disorder?" (www.AutismSpeaks.org)
- Kim, Cynthia "Accessible health care for autistic adults," (www.autismwomen'snetwork.org)
- Kuhlthau, Karen and Warfield, Marji Erickson "Transition to adult health care for youth with autism spectrum disorders," (Association of University Centers on Disabilities, www.aucd.org)
- Leeming and Lucock, "Autism: Is There a Folate Connection?" (*Journal of Inherited Metabolic Disorders,* 2009)
- Marina Sarris, "Leaving the pediatrician: charting the medical transition of youth with autism," (Interactive Autism Network at Kennedy-Krieger, 2014)
- Stahlberg, H., Soderstrom, M., and Gillberg, C. "Bipolar disorder, schizophrenia, and other psychotic disorders in adults with childhood onset AD/HD and/or autism spectrum disorders" (*Journal of Neural Transmission, 2004)*
- *Wing, Lorna and Shah, Amitta.* "A Systematic Examination of Catatonia-like Clinical Pictures in Autism Spectrum Disorders," (*International Review of Neurobiology,* 2006)

- Katharine E. Zuckerman, Alison P. Hill, Kimberly Guion, Lisa Voltolina, and Eric Fombonne, "Overweight and Obesity: Prevalence and Correlates in a Large Clinical Sample of Children with Autism Spectrum Disorder," (www.ncbi.nlm.nih.gov/pmc/articles/PMC4058357)

GLOSSARY

ABLE ACT, OR ACHIEVING A **Better Life Experience Act of 2014:** according to www.congress.gov, this act is is "to encourage and assist individuals and families in saving private funds for the purpose of supporting individuals with disabilities to maintain health, independence, and quality of life; and provide secure funding for disability-related expenses of beneficiaries with disabilities that will supplement, but not supplant, benefits provided through private insurance, Supplemental Security Income Medicaid, the beneficiary's employment, and other sources."

Adult Family Care/Adult Foster Care/AFC: a Medicaid-based program available in many American states, wherein a person with a disability lives in the home of a caregiver or caregivers, under their care. The caregiver receives a small stipend for their services.

Autism Catatonia: "a term used to refer to a cluster of behavioral features. In its extreme form, it is manifested as absence of speech (mutism), absence of movement (akinesia), and maintenance of imposed postures (catalepsy)." Dr. Lorna Wing, *British Journal of Psychiatry*, April 2000. According to Dr. Wing one in seven adolescents and young adults with autism may develop catatonia.

Benzos, Benzodiazapenes: a psychoactive medication that is often the first treatment tried in easing symptoms of autism catatonia.

Bipolar Disorder: a psychological condition wherein the patient experiences great highs and lows, depression and then periods of "mania," or highly activated, overcharged periods of almost too much energy and possibly out-of-control behavior. Bipolar can vary a lot in severity.

Day Hab/Day Habilitation: defined by the federal Center for Medicaid and Medicare Services as "provision of regularly scheduled activities in a non-residential setting, separate from the participant's private residence or other residential living arrangement, such as assistance with acquisition, retention, or improvement in self-help, socialization, and adaptive skills that enhance social development and develop skills in performing activities of daily living and community living."

Day Program, or Community-Based Day Services: daytime programs provided by state-approved organizations (service providers) for people with autism. Day programs must be provided in Home and Community Based settings and may not be provided in an institutional setting or a setting that has the qualities of an institution. Some day services include job coaching (assistance on the job) and other on-site or off-site work or community activities.

Department of Developmental Services, DDS: the state agency that oversees Medicaid waiver funding, services, support staff, and other accommodations for people with intellectual disabilities and/or developmental disabilities like autism.

Folate, Folic acid: forms of a water-soluble B vitamin. Folate occurs naturally in food, and folic acid is the synthetic form of this vitamin.

Gastroesophageal reflux disease (GERD): a painful condition that if left undiagnosed and untreated can cause significant damage to the esophagus and gastrointestinal (GI) tract.

Group Home: a housing arrangement of usually five people with disabilities, living together with some form of supervisory staff. Group homes can be privately or publicly funded, or some combination of the two. Group homes are usually created in normal neighborhoods, so as to be an integral part of a town or city but some group homes are separate communities, such as farms or other cottage industries.

Department of Health and Human Services (HHS): HHS covers many who need support services throughout the lifespan, and the AIDD (Administration of Intellectual and Developmental Disabilities) is the federal agency that deals with people on the autism spectrum.

Home and Community Based Services, HCBS: programs and housing funded through Medicaid Waivers to help keep people with developmental and/or intellectual disabilities in the community rather than in institutions.

Individualized Service Plan, ISP: the ISP team (the disabled client, service provider, daytime support people, guardians) identifies goals with the disabled adult, for housing, daytime pursuits, work, etc., and the necessary services to accomplish them. The ISP is reviewed yearly.

Institution, Institutionalization: until the recent past, it was customary to place people with intellectual disabilities, including autism, in large residences that were isolated from the rest of society. This practice is thought to be outmoded now, if not downright inhumane, and a patent denial of basic human rights of the individual to live as independently as possible within his or her community.

L-Dopa, Dopamine: according to Wikipedia, "in its pure form L-Dopa is sold as a psychoactive drug; trade names include Sinemet, Parcopa, Atamet, Stalevo, Madopar, and Prolopa. As a drug, it is used in the clinical treatment of Parkinson's disease and dopamine-responsive dystonia." It is sometimes used in treating autism catatonia.

Medicaid: the federal insurance program under the Social Security Administration that allows states to set up Home and Community Based Services for the developmentally/intellectually disabled populations (the autism community is often one such recipient).

Neuroleptic, Antipsychotic: category of drug that is frequently used in treating certain challenging autistic behaviors like aggression. Such substances and treatments should always be overseen by a qualified psychopharmacologist or psychiatrist.

PANDAs: Pediatric Autoimmune Neuropsychiatric Disorders Associated with Streptococcal Infections. People with PANDAs often exhibit obsessive-compulsive behavior and tics, sometimes seemingly "overnight." Thought to be a childhood disorder often associated with autism symptoms, there is a possibility that adults could be affected as well. Studies have been "restricted" to children, according to the NIH.

Person-Centered Planning: the philosophy and government policies created around enabling individuals with disabilities to live in their homes (not institutions) and participate in their communities to the fullest degree possible.

Section 8: federally funded housing program that provides rental assistance to eligible (limited income) people—many people with disabilities have very restricted incomes if they are living on SSI. Section 8 assistance provides eligible participants with alternative housing choices and opportunities to achieve some kind of economic independence and self-sufficiency, according to the federal Mobile Housing website. There are two kinds of vouchers for housing under Section 8: the *Mobile Voucher*, which allows the participant to get housing in any available Section 8-supported home in the country. The Mobile Voucher recipient can move anywhere to any Section 8. There is a long waiting list for Mobile Vouchers and so applicants must be sure to be on the list as soon as they turn 18.

The *Project-Based Voucher,* on the other hand, is applied to one particular building or unit, and is restricted to that unit, and does not travel with the recipient. The participant must apply to their local Housing Authorities for these particular reduced rental units.

Seizure Disorder: according to the National Institute of Mental Health: "A seizure is the physical findings or changes in behavior that occur after an episode of abnormal electrical activity in the brain." The term "seizure" is often used interchangeably with "convulsion." Convulsions occur when a person's body shakes rapidly and uncontrollably. During convulsions, the person's muscles contract and relax repeatedly. There are many different types of seizures. Some have mild symptoms without shaking.

Selective Serotonin Reuptake Inhibitor (SSRI): a class of compounds (also called serotonin-specific reuptake inhibitors) typically used as antidepressants to treat depressive disorders and anxiety disorders.

Self-Determination: an empowerment movement in the disability community and supported by the United States Government that, according to the Arc of the US, believes that "People with intellectual and/or developmental disabilities (I/DD)[1] have the same right to, and responsibilities that accompany, self-determination as everyone else. They must have opportunities, respectful support, and the authority to exert control in their lives, to self-direct their services to the extent they choose, and to advocate on their own behalf."

Service Provider: state-approved organization that provides Home-Based and/or Community residential and/or Day programs for people with developmental, intellectual, and often autism disorders.

Shared Living: a Medicaid Waiver Home-Based and Community living arrangement wherein the autistic person shares a home with a live-in fulltime caregiver, who receives a salary for his support services to the disabled client. Similar to Adult Foster Care arrangements but funded differently, under the Medicaid

Waiver administered by the state government, instead of under Medicaid itself.

Sheltered Workshop: controversial daytime setting where clients work off-site (within the Day Hab center, not out in the community). Considered by many to be outdated, isolated, and institutional in feel.

SNAP: Supplemental Nutrition Assistance Program ("food stamps"), a federal program that provides a safety net against hunger, allowing eligible participants to buy food at reduced prices

Supplemental Security Income (SSI): division of the Social Security Administration, is a benefit paid to disabled adults and children who have limited resources and income.

Stims: self-stimulatory behavior, sometimes called stereotypical behavior.

Transition to Adulthood: federal program under the IDEA, Individuals with Disabilities Education Act, requiring school systems and state agencies to plan with the disabled student his or her future as an adult, post-twenty-two. Transition to Adulthood meetings should begin at age sixteen.

Turning twenty-two: federal program that stipulates that a disabled person's public education ends at age twenty-two and he moves into the adult services system.

Waiver, Medicaid Waiver, Waiver Funding: according to the Arc of the US, "states may submit applications to the federal Center for Medicaid Services for approval to waive certain requirements of the Medicaid program in order to provide Home and Community-Based Services (HCBS) as an alternative to providing those services in institutional settings, such as nursing homes and intermediate care facilities for individuals with intellectual and developmental disabilities (ICF/IDD)." These waivers are permitted by Section 1915(c) of the Social Security Act and are called 1915(c) waivers. Many individuals with intellectual and developmental disabilities receive HCBS through1915(c) waivers that enable them to live in their own homes.